Thyroid Health Revitalized

Restoring Balance for Lasting Thyroid Well-Being

BY

Dr. Luna Jefferson

Copyright

No part of this book should be copied, reproduced without the author's permission © 2023

TABLE OF CONTENT

INTRODUCTION

Introduction to the thyroid gland

The thyroid gland, a small butterfly-shaped organ nestled in the neck just below the Adam's apple, plays a pivotal role in maintaining the body's delicate balance and overall well-being. This unassuming gland is often underestimated in its significance, yet it serves as a regulatory powerhouse, influencing numerous physiological processes.

At its core, the thyroid is the body's metabolic master, orchestrating energy production and consumption. It accomplishes this through the secretion of thyroid hormones—chiefly thyroxine (T4) and triiodothyronine (T3). These hormones act as messengers, traversing the bloodstream to reach virtually every cell in the body. Once there, they exert control over metabolism, affecting how the body uses energy derived from food.

The thyroid's importance extends beyond metabolism; it also wields influence over temperature regulation, heart rate, and the maintenance of healthy skin, hair, and nails. This gland acts as a silent conductor, orchestrating a symphony of bodily functions to ensure harmony and optimal performance.

An intricate feedback loop involving the pituitary gland and the hypothalamus ensures that the thyroid operates in synchrony with the body's needs. When levels of thyroid hormones drop, the hypothalamus signals the pituitary gland to release thyroid-stimulating hormone (TSH), prompting the thyroid to ramp up hormone production. Conversely, elevated hormone levels trigger a decrease in TSH release, maintaining a delicate equilibrium.

The consequences of thyroid dysfunction can be profound, ranging from subtle changes in energy levels to more severe conditions such as hypothyroidism or hyperthyroidism. As we delve into the intricacies of the thyroid in this book, it becomes clear that understanding its role is paramount to comprehending the complexities of thyroid disorders. By demystifying the functions of this seemingly modest gland, we empower ourselves to navigate the challenges of thyroid health, paving the way for informed decisions and improved overall well-being.

Basic anatomy and function of the thyroid

The thyroid gland, a marvel of biological engineering, is a small, butterfly-shaped organ situated at the base of the neck, just above the collarbone. This unassuming structure belies its profound impact on the body's intricate regulatory systems. The thyroid consists of two lobes, resembling wings, connected by a narrow band of tissue known as the isthmus.

Within its cellular framework, the thyroid harbors numerous follicles, small sac-like structures that house a protein-rich colloid. It is within these follicles that the thyroid's essential work takes place. The gland's primary function revolves around the synthesis and secretion of thyroid hormones—thyroxine (T4) and triiodothyronine (T3). These hormones are synthesized from iodine, an essential mineral derived from the diet, and tyrosine, an amino acid.

The synthesis process begins with the uptake of iodine from the bloodstream by the thyroid follicular cells. The iodine is then incorporated into the amino acid tyrosine within the colloid, resulting in the formation of T3 and T4. Once synthesized, these hormones are stored within the follicles until the body signals a need for their release.

The release of thyroid hormones is carefully orchestrated by the thyroid-stimulating hormone (TSH) secreted by the pituitary gland. TSH stimulates the thyroid to release T3 and T4 into the bloodstream, where they travel to target cells throughout the body. The metabolic effects of these hormones are far-reaching, influencing energy production, growth, and the functioning of various organs and tissues.

The thyroid's finely tuned control over metabolism and energy balance highlights its central role in maintaining homeostasis. Any disruption in this delicate equilibrium can lead to thyroid disorders, impacting not only the gland itself but also cascading effects on overall health. As we delve into the complexities of thyroid anatomy and function in this book, a deeper appreciation for the thyroid's pivotal role in our well-being emerges, guiding our understanding of thyroid-related conditions and their management.

Dispelling common myths and misconceptions

Dispelling Common Myths and Misconceptions About the Thyroid

The thyroid gland, with its intricate role in regulating metabolism and overall health, has become the subject of numerous myths and misconceptions that, unfortunately, can contribute to confusion and misinformation. It is essential to dispel these myths to foster a more accurate understanding of thyroid health.

One prevalent myth is that thyroid disorders only affect women. While it's true that women are more prone to thyroid conditions, men can also experience them. Hormonal fluctuations, autoimmune factors, and genetic predispositions contribute to thyroid disorders, affecting individuals of any gender.

Another misconception is that thyroid disorders are always accompanied by noticeable symptoms. In reality, some thyroid conditions can be asymptomatic or present with subtle signs that may be overlooked. Regular check-ups and awareness of risk factors are crucial for early detection and intervention.

A commonly misunderstood concept is that weight gain or loss is the sole indicator of thyroid dysfunction. While thyroid disorders can indeed influence weight, they manifest in a spectrum of symptoms, including fatigue, changes in skin and hair texture, and alterations in mood and cognitive function. A comprehensive understanding of these symptoms is vital for accurate diagnosis.

There's also a belief that thyroid disorders are always permanent. In truth, some conditions, such as thyroiditis, may be transient and reversible. Proper diagnosis and management can lead to the restoration of thyroid function in certain cases.

Lastly, the idea that thyroid health is solely dependent on iodine intake oversimplifies the complex interplay of factors affecting the thyroid. While iodine is crucial for thyroid hormone synthesis, an excessive intake can be as detrimental as a deficiency. A balanced diet, proper medical care, and lifestyle factors contribute collectively to thyroid health.

By dispelling these common myths and misconceptions, we pave the way for a more informed and nuanced understanding of thyroid health. This awareness empowers individuals to make informed decisions, seek timely medical advice, and engage in proactive measures to maintain a healthy thyroid and overall well-being.

CHAPTER ONE

Thyroid Virus Triggers

Understanding Thyroid Virus Triggers

Thyroid disorders can often be traced back to various triggers, and among them, viral infections emerge as significant contributors. Viruses, microscopic entities that invade cells and replicate within them, can provoke immune responses that, in turn, impact the thyroid gland. The relationship between viruses and thyroid dysfunction is complex and multifaceted.

One notable viral trigger is the Epstein-Barr virus (EBV), a member of the herpesvirus family. Studies suggest a connection between EBV and autoimmune thyroid disorders, particularly Hashimoto's disease. The virus can initiate an autoimmune response, causing the immune system to mistakenly attack the thyroid tissue. This inflammatory process can lead to the gradual destruction of thyroid cells, impairing the gland's function.

Another viral player in thyroid disorders is the human immunodeficiency virus (HIV). While not a direct cause, HIV can indirectly affect the thyroid by compromising the immune system. This immune dysfunction may trigger thyroiditis or exacerbate existing thyroid conditions.

Certain respiratory viruses, such as influenza and respiratory syncytial virus (RSV), have also been implicated in thyroid dysfunction. The immune response mounted against these viruses can induce inflammation and potentially lead to thyroiditis, disrupting the normal functioning of the thyroid.

Furthermore, research suggests a correlation between viral infections and the development of Graves' disease, an autoimmune disorder characterized by overactive thyroid function. Viruses may act as environmental triggers, influencing the onset of Graves' disease in genetically predisposed individuals.

Understanding these viral triggers is crucial for both prevention and management. Practicing good hygiene, especially during viral seasons, and maintaining a healthy immune system through vaccination and lifestyle choices can help reduce the risk of viral infections impacting the thyroid. Additionally, individuals with existing thyroid conditions should be vigilant about monitoring their thyroid health during and after viral illnesses to ensure timely intervention and appropriate management.

Exploring factors that can trigger thyroid disorders

Thyroid disorders, encompassing conditions like hypothyroidism, hyperthyroidism, and autoimmune diseases, can arise from a complex interplay of genetic, environmental, and lifestyle factors. Understanding these triggers is essential for both prevention and effective management of thyroid-related conditions.

Genetic Predisposition: A family history of thyroid disorders increases the likelihood of an individual developing similar conditions. Certain genetic variations can make individuals more susceptible to thyroid dysfunction, emphasizing the importance of genetic factors in the risk profile.

Autoimmune Factors: Autoimmune thyroid disorders, such as Hashimoto's disease and Graves' disease, occur when the immune system mistakenly attacks the thyroid gland. Genetic predisposition, combined with environmental triggers like infections or stress, can contribute to the development of these conditions.

Iodine Intake: While iodine is essential for thyroid hormone production, both deficiency and excess can be problematic. In regions with iodine deficiency, the risk of hypothyroidism increases, while excessive iodine intake, often from supplements or certain foods, can contribute to hyperthyroidism.

Pregnancy and Hormonal Changes: Pregnancy and hormonal fluctuations, such as those during menopause, can impact thyroid function. Postpartum thyroiditis, characterized by temporary thyroid dysfunction after childbirth, is an example of how hormonal changes can trigger thyroid disorders.

Stress and Lifestyle Factors: Chronic stress can adversely affect the immune system and contribute to inflammation, potentially triggering or exacerbating thyroid disorders. Additionally, lifestyle factors such as poor diet, lack of exercise, and inadequate sleep can influence thyroid health.

Environmental Toxins: Exposure to environmental toxins like pollutants and certain chemicals may disrupt thyroid function. Endocrine-disrupting chemicals can interfere with the production and regulation of thyroid hormones, contributing to thyroid dysfunction.

Radiation Exposure: Radiation, whether from medical treatments or environmental sources, poses a risk to the thyroid. Radiation therapy for head and neck cancers, for example, may inadvertently impact thyroid function.

By recognizing and addressing these triggers, individuals can adopt preventive measures and make informed lifestyle choices to support thyroid health. Regular monitoring and seeking medical advice for potential risk factors can contribute to early detection and effective management of thyroid disorders.

Understanding the Role of Viruses in Thyroid Dysfunction

Viruses, microscopic entities capable of infecting cells and altering their function, have been identified as potential contributors to thyroid dysfunction. The intricate relationship between viral infections and the thyroid involves a complex interplay of immune responses, genetic factors, and environmental triggers.

Autoimmune Response: Viral infections can trigger an autoimmune response, where the immune system, in its attempt to eliminate the virus, mistakenly attacks the thyroid tissue. This phenomenon is particularly relevant in autoimmune thyroid disorders such as Hashimoto's disease. The immune system, sensitized by the viral infection, may recognize thyroid antigens as foreign, leading to an ongoing autoimmune attack on the thyroid gland.

Inflammation and Thyroiditis: Certain viruses can induce inflammation, directly affecting the thyroid gland and leading to a condition known as thyroiditis. Inflammation can disrupt the normal functioning of the thyroid, impacting hormone production and release. This inflammatory response may be acute or chronic, contributing to various forms of thyroiditis, including subacute thyroiditis and chronic lymphocytic thyroiditis.

Direct Viral Invasion: In some cases, viruses may directly invade thyroid cells, disrupting their structure and function. This direct invasion can impair the synthesis and release of thyroid hormones, leading to thyroid dysfunction. While less common, direct viral effects on the thyroid have been observed in certain viral infections.

Immune Modulation: Viruses can modulate the immune system, influencing the balance between proinflammatory and anti-inflammatory responses. This immune modulation can affect the delicate equilibrium required for proper thyroid function. Imbalances in the immune system, triggered by viral infections, may contribute to the development or exacerbation of thyroid disorders.

Environmental Triggers: Viral infections can act as environmental triggers, particularly in individuals genetically predisposed to thyroid dysfunction. The combination of genetic susceptibility and exposure to specific viruses may increase the risk of developing thyroid disorders.

Recognizing the role of viruses in thyroid dysfunction underscores the importance of a comprehensive approach to thyroid health. Prevention through vaccination, managing viral infections promptly, and addressing autoimmune responses are critical aspects of preserving thyroid function. Individuals with a history of viral infections or autoimmune conditions should be vigilant about monitoring their thyroid health, seeking medical attention for early detection and appropriate management.

CHAPTER TWO

How the Thyroid Virus Works

The relationship between viruses and thyroid function involves a sophisticated interplay of biological processes, immune responses, and the delicate balance that sustains thyroid health. The thyroid virus, often implicated in the context of autoimmune thyroid disorders, operates through intricate mechanisms that impact the thyroid gland on multiple levels.

Triggering Autoimmune Responses: In some cases, viruses can act as triggers for autoimmune thyroid disorders by initiating an immune response. When the body encounters a viral infection, the immune system mounts a defense to eliminate the virus. However, in susceptible individuals, this immune response may become misdirected, leading to the production of antibodies that mistakenly target the thyroid tissue. This phenomenon, known as molecular mimicry, can result in an autoimmune attack on the thyroid.

Interference with Thyroid Cells: Viruses may directly invade thyroid cells, disrupting their structure and function. The virus can exploit the cellular machinery of the thyroid cells for replication, potentially leading to cell damage and dysfunction. This direct interference can impair the synthesis and release of thyroid hormones, influencing the overall balance of the endocrine system.

Induction of Inflammation: Many viral infections stimulate an inflammatory response in the body. This inflammation can extend to the thyroid gland, causing thyroiditis—a condition characterized by inflammation of the thyroid. Inflammatory processes can hinder the normal functioning of the thyroid, impacting hormone production and release. This can manifest as temporary thyroid dysfunction or, in some cases, contribute to chronic thyroid conditions.

Modulation of Immune System: Viruses have the ability to modulate the immune system, influencing the delicate balance between pro-inflammatory and anti-inflammatory responses. This modulation can have profound effects on the immune cells that regulate thyroid function. Imbalances in immune modulation, triggered by viral infections, may contribute to the development or exacerbation of thyroid disorders.

Understanding how the thyroid virus operates is crucial for unraveling the complexities of thyroid dysfunction. By deciphering these mechanisms, researchers and healthcare professionals can develop targeted interventions and therapeutic strategies to mitigate the impact of viral triggers on thyroid health. This knowledge also empowers individuals to adopt preventive measures and make informed choices for their overall well-being.

In-depth Look at the Mechanisms Behind Thyroid Virus Infections

Thyroid virus infections involve intricate molecular and immunological processes that can disrupt the finely tuned balance of the thyroid gland. One key mechanism is the virus's ability to exploit host cells for replication. The virus may infiltrate thyroid cells, utilizing their machinery to replicate and propagate, leading to cellular damage and dysfunction.

Furthermore, certain viruses trigger an autoimmune response through molecular mimicry. This occurs when viral proteins structurally resemble thyroid proteins. The immune system, in its attempt to eradicate the virus, may inadvertently target the thyroid tissue, inducing an autoimmune attack. This phenomenon is particularly relevant in autoimmune thyroid disorders like Hashimoto's disease and Graves' disease.

The induction of inflammation is another crucial mechanism. Viral infections often provoke an inflammatory response, and when this inflammation extends to the thyroid gland, it can result in thyroiditis. Inflammatory processes can impair the normal functioning of thyroid cells, affecting hormone synthesis and release.

Understanding these mechanisms is pivotal for developing targeted interventions and therapeutic approaches to mitigate the impact of thyroid virus infections. Researchers delve into the molecular intricacies of viral interactions with thyroid cells to unravel potential points of intervention, aiming to preserve thyroid health and prevent the onset or progression of thyroid disorders.

Impact on thyroid function and overall health

The impact of thyroid virus infections extends beyond the immediate infection itself, profoundly influencing both thyroid function and overall health. Viruses can disrupt the intricate balance of thyroid hormones, compromising the gland's ability to regulate metabolism, energy production, and various physiological processes. This disruption often leads to thyroid dysfunction, with consequences ranging from subtle imbalances to more severe conditions like hypothyroidism or hyperthyroidism.

In the context of autoimmune thyroid disorders, the immune response triggered by viral infections can result in persistent inflammation and damage to thyroid tissue. This, in turn, contributes to chronic conditions such as Hashimoto's disease or Graves' disease, where the immune system mistakenly attacks the thyroid.

Thyroid dysfunction has far-reaching implications for overall health. The thyroid hormones play a crucial role in maintaining homeostasis, influencing the function of organs and tissues throughout the body. Disruptions in thyroid function can manifest as fatigue, weight fluctuations, mood disturbances, and impaired cognitive function, impacting an individual's quality of life.

Beyond the immediate physiological effects, the systemic impact of thyroid virus infections underscores the importance of timely intervention, comprehensive management, and preventive measures. Understanding these interconnected dynamics is essential for healthcare professionals and individuals alike to address not only the viral infection but also its potential long-term consequences on thyroid health and overall well-being.

CHAPTER THREE

Your Thyroid's True Purpose

The thyroid, a seemingly modest butterfly-shaped gland situated in the neck, holds profound significance in maintaining the delicate balance of the body. Its true purpose goes beyond its small size, as it plays a central role in orchestrating key physiological functions essential for overall well-being.

At its core, the thyroid serves as the body's metabolic maestro, regulating the rate at which cells convert food into energy. This vital function is accomplished through the production and secretion of thyroid hormones—chiefly thyroxine (T4) and triiodothyronine (T3). These hormones act as messengers, influencing virtually every cell and organ in the body to ensure a harmonious and efficient metabolism.

In addition to its metabolic role, the thyroid contributes significantly to temperature regulation. Thyroid hormones help maintain the body's core temperature, ensuring that various biochemical reactions occur optimally. This thermoregulatory function is crucial for sustaining normal bodily functions and preventing temperature-related complications.

The thyroid's influence extends to the cardiovascular system, where it regulates heart rate and blood pressure. By modulating the sensitivity of cells to adrenaline and controlling the contraction strength of the heart muscle, the thyroid ensures a steady cardiovascular rhythm.

Beyond these fundamental functions, the thyroid is intricately involved in the growth and development of tissues and organs, particularly during childhood and adolescence. It influences bone development, neural maturation, and the overall physical and cognitive growth of an individual.

In essence, the true purpose of the thyroid is to act as a master regulator, fine-tuning the body's metabolism, temperature, and growth processes. Its harmonious functioning is crucial for maintaining homeostasis and ensuring that all physiological systems work in tandem.

Understanding the thyroid's true purpose underscores its significance in overall health. An imbalance in thyroid function can have far-reaching consequences, affecting energy levels, mood, and various bodily functions. By appreciating the thyroid's multifaceted role, individuals can recognize the importance of maintaining thyroid health through proper nutrition, lifestyle choices, and regular medical check-ups.

A Detailed Exploration of the Thyroid's Role in the Body

The thyroid, a small but mighty gland located in the neck, exerts a profound influence on the body's intricate web of functions. Its role extends far beyond its size, as it serves as a master regulator, orchestrating key processes that contribute to overall health and well-being.

Metabolic Control: At the heart of the thyroid's responsibilities is the regulation of metabolism. The thyroid produces and releases hormones—thyroxine (T4) and triiodothyronine (T3)—that play a pivotal role in determining how cells utilize energy derived from food. By influencing metabolic rate, the thyroid ensures that the body efficiently converts nutrients into energy, maintaining a delicate balance.

Thermoregulation: The thyroid also contributes to the body's temperature regulation. Thyroid hormones influence heat production and dissipation, helping to maintain a constant core temperature. This thermoregulatory function is essential for sustaining enzymatic reactions and cellular processes at optimal rates.

Cardiovascular Harmony: Through its influence on the cardiovascular system, the thyroid modulates heart rate and blood pressure. Thyroid hormones affect the responsiveness of cells to adrenaline and control the strength of the heart's contractions. This regulation ensures a steady and efficient circulation of blood throughout the body.

Growth and Development: Particularly crucial during periods of growth and development, the thyroid impacts the maturation of tissues and organs. It plays a vital role in bone development, neural maturation, and the maintenance of overall physical and cognitive growth, especially in childhood and adolescence.

Neurological and Cognitive Functions: Thyroid hormones have a significant impact on neurological and cognitive functions. They contribute to the development and maintenance of the central nervous system, influencing mood, memory, and concentration.

In essence, the thyroid's detailed role encompasses a symphony of functions crucial for maintaining homeostasis. Imbalances in thyroid function can lead to a cascade of effects, impacting energy levels, body temperature, cardiovascular health, and overall growth and development. A nuanced understanding of the thyroid's multifaceted role underscores the importance of prioritizing thyroid health through regular monitoring, proper nutrition, and lifestyle choices.

How the Thyroid Contributes to Maintaining Balance and Homeostasis

The thyroid gland stands as a sentinel of balance within the human body, contributing significantly to the maintenance of homeostasis, a state of internal equilibrium necessary for optimal physiological functioning. Its multifaceted functions act as crucial regulators, ensuring that various systems work in tandem to sustain overall health.

Metabolic Equilibrium: One of the primary roles of the thyroid is to regulate metabolism, the process by which the body converts food into energy. Through the secretion of thyroid hormones, the gland fine-tunes the metabolic rate, balancing energy production and consumption. This metabolic equilibrium is vital for preventing fluctuations in weight, sustaining energy levels, and supporting the efficient functioning of cells.

Temperature Regulation: The thyroid plays a pivotal role in thermoregulation, maintaining the body's core temperature within a narrow range. By influencing heat production and dissipation, thyroid hormones contribute to temperature homeostasis. This ensures that enzymatic reactions and cellular processes occur optimally, preventing disruptions that could arise from temperature extremes.

Cardiovascular Harmony: Thyroid hormones intricately influence the cardiovascular system, regulating heart rate and blood pressure. This cardiovascular harmony is essential for ensuring adequate blood flow to tissues and organs. By modulating the responsiveness of cells to adrenaline and controlling the strength of heart contractions, the thyroid contributes to maintaining a steady and efficient circulation.

Neuroendocrine Communication: The thyroid engages in complex communication with the nervous system, impacting neurological functions and cognitive processes. It influences mood, memory, and concentration, contributing to the delicate balance of mental and emotional well-being.

Growth and Development: Especially crucial during periods of growth and development, the thyroid ensures equilibrium in the maturation of tissues and organs. It supports bone development, neural maturation, and overall physical and cognitive growth, promoting a harmonious progression from childhood through adolescence.

In essence, the thyroid's contribution to maintaining balance and homeostasis is pervasive, influencing fundamental aspects of metabolism, temperature regulation, cardiovascular function, neurological health, and growth. Recognizing the integral role of the thyroid in these processes underscores the importance of preserving its health through proactive measures, regular monitoring, and a holistic approach to well-being.

CHAPTER FOUR

Your Symptoms and Conditions

Understanding the symptoms and conditions associated with thyroid dysfunction is pivotal for individuals seeking to maintain their overall well-being. The thyroid, a small yet influential gland, can manifest imbalances through a spectrum of symptoms and conditions that vary in severity and presentation.

Common Symptoms: Recognizing the subtle signs of thyroid dysfunction is crucial. Fatigue, weight changes, mood swings, and alterations in skin, hair, and nail texture are often early indicators. Individuals might experience difficulty concentrating, fluctuations in body temperature, and changes in bowel habits. Sensitivity to cold or heat, muscle weakness, and joint pain can also be associated symptoms.

Hypothyroidism: Hypothyroidism, characterized by an underactive thyroid, can lead to a cluster of symptoms such as fatigue, weight gain, cold intolerance, and depression. Skin may become dry, and hair and nails brittle. Constipation and menstrual irregularities may also occur. Left untreated, hypothyroidism can have widespread effects on the body, affecting cardiovascular, metabolic, and cognitive functions.

Hyperthyroidism: Conversely, hyperthyroidism, or an overactive thyroid, can present with symptoms like weight loss, increased heart rate, anxiety, and heat intolerance. Individuals may experience muscle weakness, trembling hands, and changes in bowel habits. The eyes may exhibit signs of Graves' disease, a common cause of hyperthyroidism, with bulging or irritation.

Autoimmune Thyroid Disorders: Conditions such as Hashimoto's disease and Graves' disease are autoimmune disorders where the immune system mistakenly attacks the thyroid. Hashimoto's often leads to hypothyroidism, while Graves' results in hyperthyroidism. Both can present with additional symptoms such as goiter, where the thyroid gland becomes enlarged.

Navigating the landscape of thyroid health involves vigilance and awareness of these symptoms. Timely consultation with healthcare professionals, comprehensive diagnostic tests, and regular monitoring are crucial for accurate diagnosis and effective management. By understanding the nuances of symptoms and conditions associated with thyroid dysfunction, individuals can take proactive steps toward preserving their thyroid health and overall quality of life.

Discussion of Common Symptoms Associated with Thyroid Disorders

Thyroid disorders, encompassing conditions like hypothyroidism and hyperthyroidism, often manifest through a range of symptoms that can significantly impact an individual's well-being. Recognizing these common symptoms is key to early detection and effective management of thyroid-related conditions.

Fatigue: Persistent fatigue is a hallmark symptom of thyroid disorders, whether it be hypothyroidism or hyperthyroidism. Individuals may experience a profound and unrelenting sense of tiredness that goes beyond normal fatigue.

Weight Changes: Fluctuations in weight are common indicators of thyroid dysfunction. Hypothyroidism is often associated with weight gain, while hyperthyroidism may lead to unexplained weight loss.

Mood Swings: Thyroid disorders can influence mood and emotional well-being. Hypothyroidism is linked to symptoms like depression, anxiety, and irritability, while hyperthyroidism may cause heightened anxiety and restlessness.

Changes in Skin, Hair, and Nails: Dry skin, brittle nails, and hair loss are frequently observed in individuals with thyroid disorders. Changes in the texture and appearance of skin, hair, and nails are often indicative of an underlying thyroid imbalance.

Temperature Sensitivity: Thyroid hormones play a crucial role in regulating body temperature. Individuals with hypothyroidism may feel excessively cold, while those with hyperthyroidism may experience heightened sensitivity to heat.

Heart Rate and Palpitations: Cardiovascular symptoms are common in thyroid disorders. Hypothyroidism may lead to a slowed heart rate, while hyperthyroidism can cause an elevated heart rate and palpitations.

Digestive Issues: Changes in bowel habits, including constipation or diarrhea, are frequently associated with thyroid dysfunction. The thyroid's influence on the digestive system can lead to disruptions in normal gastrointestinal function.

Recognizing these symptoms and their variations is essential for seeking timely medical attention. Comprehensive diagnostic tests, including thyroid function tests, help healthcare professionals accurately diagnose the specific thyroid disorder and tailor an appropriate treatment plan. Early intervention and management can significantly improve quality of life for individuals living with thyroid disorders.

Managing Thyroid-Related Symptoms

Effective management of thyroid-related symptoms involves a multifaceted approach that considers the specific condition, its underlying causes, and the individual's overall health. Here's a detailed guide on managing various symptoms associated with thyroid disorders:

Fatigue:

1. Balanced Diet: Ensure a nutrient-rich diet with a mix of carbohydrates, proteins, and healthy fats to sustain energy levels.

2. Regular Exercise: Engage in moderate exercise to improve overall energy and combat fatigue. Avoid excessive exertion, especially in cases of hyperthyroidism.

Weight Changes:

1. Healthy Eating Habits: Adopt a well-balanced diet, emphasizing whole foods and portion control. Consult a nutritionist for personalized guidance.
2. Regular Physical Activity: Incorporate regular exercise, including both aerobic and strength training, to support metabolism and weight management.

Mood Swings:

1. Stress Management: Practice stress-reducing techniques such as meditation, deep breathing, or yoga to alleviate anxiety and mood swings.
2. Therapeutic Support: Consider counseling or therapy for emotional support and coping strategies.

Changes in Skin, Hair, and Nails:

1. Hydration: Ensure proper hydration to support skin health. Use moisturizers to alleviate dry skin.
2. Hair and Nail Care: Adopt a gentle hair care routine, and consider biotin supplements for hair and nail strength.

Temperature Sensitivity:

1. Layer Clothing: Dress in layers to adjust to temperature fluctuations.
2. Maintain Room Temperature: Keep indoor spaces at a comfortable temperature, especially for those sensitive to cold.

Heart Rate and Palpitations:

1. Limit Stimulants: Reduce caffeine and stimulant intake to minimize palpitations.
2. Medication Adjustment: Work closely with healthcare providers to adjust thyroid medication dosage for optimal control.

Digestive Issues:

1. Dietary Fiber: Consume a fiber-rich diet to regulate bowel movements.
2. Hydration: Drink plenty of water to prevent constipation.

Specific Conditions:

1. Hypothyroidism: Adherence to thyroid medication is crucial. Regular monitoring of thyroid levels and adjustments to medication dosage are common management strategies.
2. Hyperthyroidism: Antithyroid medications, radioactive iodine, or thyroidectomy may be recommended based on the severity of hyperthyroidism.

General Tips for Thyroid Health:

1. Regular Check-ups: Schedule regular thyroid function tests to monitor hormone levels.

2. Medication Compliance: Adhere to prescribed medications and attend follow-up appointments.

3. Lifestyle Modifications: Adopt a healthy lifestyle with regular exercise, a balanced diet, and sufficient sleep.

Individualized management plans are essential, and consultation with healthcare professionals, including endocrinologists and nutritionists, is highly recommended. Tailoring strategies to specific symptoms and the underlying thyroid condition ensures a comprehensive and effective approach to managing thyroid-related symptoms.

An Overview of Various Thyroid-Related Conditions

Thyroid-related conditions encompass a spectrum of disorders that affect the function and structure of the thyroid gland, a crucial component of the endocrine system. Understanding these conditions is vital for individuals and healthcare professionals alike to navigate the complexities of thyroid health.

1. Hypothyroidism: Characterized by an underactive thyroid, hypothyroidism occurs when the gland does not produce sufficient thyroid hormones. Common symptoms include fatigue, weight gain, cold intolerance, and depression. Hashimoto's disease, an autoimmune condition, is a leading cause of hypothyroidism.

2. Hyperthyroidism: In contrast, hyperthyroidism results from an overactive thyroid, leading to an excess of thyroid hormones. Symptoms may include weight loss, increased heart rate, anxiety, and heat intolerance. Graves' disease, an autoimmune disorder, is a prevalent cause of hyperthyroidism.

3. Hashimoto's Disease: An autoimmune disorder, Hashimoto's disease is the most common cause of hypothyroidism. The immune system mistakenly attacks the thyroid, leading to inflammation and gradual destruction of thyroid tissue.

4. Graves' Disease: Another autoimmune condition, Graves' disease causes the immune system to stimulate the thyroid excessively, resulting in hyperthyroidism. It is often characterized by symptoms such as bulging eyes (exophthalmos), weight loss, and goiter.

5. Thyroid Nodules: Thyroid nodules are abnormal growths or lumps within the thyroid gland. While most nodules are benign, some may be cancerous. The presence of nodules may lead to changes in thyroid function or cause discomfort.

6. Thyroid Cancer: Although relatively rare, thyroid cancer can occur. It is often characterized by the presence of nodules, changes in voice, difficulty swallowing, or swelling in the neck. Early detection and treatment are crucial for favorable outcomes.

7. Thyroiditis: Inflammation of the thyroid, known as thyroiditis, can cause temporary disruptions in thyroid function. Subtypes include Hashimoto's thyroiditis, postpartum thyroiditis, and subacute thyroiditis.

Understanding the nuances of these thyroid-related conditions empowers individuals to recognize symptoms, seek timely medical attention, and engage in informed discussions with healthcare professionals. Early detection, accurate diagnosis, and appropriate management are key factors in promoting optimal thyroid health and overall well-being.

CHAPTER FIVE

Thyroid Cancer

Thyroid cancer, though relatively uncommon compared to other cancers, is a significant health concern characterized by the abnormal growth of cells in the thyroid gland. Nestled in the neck, the thyroid plays a crucial role in regulating metabolism through the production of hormones. When normal thyroid cells undergo malignant transformation, they give rise to thyroid cancer.

There are several types of thyroid cancer, with papillary and follicular carcinomas being the most prevalent. Medullary and anaplastic carcinomas are rarer but more aggressive forms. Risk factors for thyroid cancer include a family history of the disease, exposure to radiation, and certain genetic conditions.

Thyroid cancer often presents as a painless lump or nodule in the neck, but symptoms may vary depending on the specific type and stage of the cancer. Diagnostic tools include imaging studies, such as ultrasound and biopsy, to confirm the presence of cancerous cells.

Treatment approaches encompass surgery, radioactive iodine therapy, and, in advanced cases, external beam radiation. The prognosis for thyroid cancer is generally favorable, particularly with early detection and appropriate intervention. A comprehensive understanding of thyroid cancer is vital for effective management and underscores the importance of regular screenings for those at risk.

Understanding Thyroid Cancer, Its Types, and Risk Factors

Thyroid cancer is a relatively rare but significant malignancy that originates in the thyroid gland, a small butterfly-shaped organ located at the base of the neck. Comprehending the intricacies of thyroid cancer involves exploring its types, recognizing potential risk factors, and understanding its impact on health.

Types of Thyroid Cancer:

1. Papillary Carcinoma: The most prevalent form, accounting for about 80% of cases, papillary carcinoma arises from follicular cells and generally has a favorable prognosis. It often presents as a painless lump or nodule in the thyroid.

2. Follicular Carcinoma: Making up approximately 10-15% of thyroid cancer cases, follicular carcinoma originates in the thyroid's follicular cells. While it tends to have a good prognosis, it may have a higher likelihood of spreading to blood vessels.

3. Medullary Carcinoma: Derived from thyroid C cells, medullary carcinoma constitutes about 4-5% of thyroid cancers. It may be associated with genetic syndromes and has a higher tendency to spread to lymph nodes.

4. Anaplastic Carcinoma: Though rare, anaplastic carcinoma is an aggressive and fast-growing form of thyroid cancer. It often presents in advanced stages and carries a less favorable prognosis.

Risk Factors:

1. Gender and Age: Thyroid cancer is more prevalent in women than men, and the risk increases with age, particularly after the age of 40.

2. Radiation Exposure: Exposure to ionizing radiation, whether from medical treatments, environmental sources, or certain workplace conditions, is a well-established risk factor for thyroid cancer.

3. Family History: A family history of thyroid cancer or certain genetic conditions, such as familial medullary thyroid cancer or multiple endocrine neoplasia, elevates the risk.

4. Iodine Deficiency or Excess: While iodine deficiency is linked to an increased risk of certain thyroid conditions, excessive iodine intake can also contribute to thyroid cancer, particularly in predisposed individuals.

5. Genetic Factors: Specific genetic mutations, such as those associated with the RET proto-oncogene, increase susceptibility to medullary thyroid cancer.

Understanding these types and risk factors is pivotal for early detection and effective management of thyroid cancer. Regular screenings, particularly for individuals with known risk factors, can aid in timely diagnosis and intervention, contributing to better outcomes and quality of life for those affected by thyroid cancer.

Diagnosis and Treatment Options for Thyroid Cancer

Diagnosis:

1. Physical Examination and Medical History: Initial assessment involves a thorough examination of the neck to detect any abnormalities or palpable nodules. A detailed medical history is obtained, including family history and exposure to risk factors.

2. Imaging Studies: Imaging tools such as ultrasound, CT scans, or MRI are employed to visualize the thyroid gland and assess the extent of the tumor. These studies aid in determining the size, location, and potential spread of the cancer.

3. Fine Needle Aspiration (FNA) Biopsy: A crucial diagnostic tool, FNA biopsy involves extracting a small tissue sample from the thyroid nodule using a thin needle. The sample is then examined under a microscope to identify cancerous cells and determine the specific type of thyroid cancer.

4. Blood Tests: Blood tests, including thyroid function tests and measurement of specific tumor markers,

provide additional information about the thyroid's overall function and the presence of certain proteins associated with thyroid cancer.

Treatment Options:

1. Surgery:
  - Thyroidectomy: The primary treatment for thyroid cancer involves surgical removal of the thyroid gland. The extent of surgery depends on the type and stage of the cancer.
  - Lymph Node Dissection: In cases where cancer has spread to nearby lymph nodes, surgical removal of affected nodes may be necessary.

2. Radioactive Iodine Therapy (RAI):
  - RAI is often recommended after surgery to eliminate any remaining thyroid tissue or cancer cells. Thyroid cells have a unique ability to absorb iodine, making this treatment effective in targeting residual cancer cells.

3. Hormone Replacement Therapy:
  - Following thyroidectomy, patients require lifelong hormone replacement therapy with synthetic thyroid hormones (levothyroxine) to maintain normal hormonal levels and prevent hypothyroidism.

4. External Beam Radiation Therapy:

- In cases where thyroid cancer is more advanced or not responsive to RAI, external beam radiation therapy may be employed to target cancer cells with high-energy beams.

5. Targeted Therapies and Chemotherapy:
  - For aggressive forms of thyroid cancer, targeted therapies and chemotherapy may be considered to impede cancer cell growth and metastasis.

6. Clinical Trials:
  - Participation in clinical trials may be an option for individuals with advanced or refractory thyroid cancer, providing access to novel treatments and therapies.

A multidisciplinary approach involving endocrinologists, surgeons, oncologists, and other specialists is crucial for devising an individualized treatment plan. Regular follow-up and monitoring are essential to track the response to treatment and address any potential complications or recurrence of thyroid cancer.

CHAPTER SIX

Hyperthyroidism

Hyperthyroidism is a medical condition characterized by an overactive thyroid gland, resulting in excessive production and release of thyroid hormones into the bloodstream. The thyroid gland, situated in the neck, plays a pivotal role in regulating metabolism and energy expenditure by producing hormones such as thyroxine (T4) and triiodothyronine (T3).

In hyperthyroidism, the thyroid gland becomes hyperfunctional, leading to an imbalance in hormone levels. This excess of thyroid hormones accelerates metabolic processes throughout the body, impacting various physiological functions. The most common cause of hyperthyroidism is Graves' disease, an autoimmune disorder where the immune system erroneously stimulates the thyroid to produce more hormones.

Understanding the symptoms of hyperthyroidism is crucial for early detection and management. Common signs include:

1. Weight Loss: Despite an increased appetite, individuals with hyperthyroidism often experience unintentional weight loss.

2. Increased Heart Rate: The excess thyroid hormones can elevate the heart rate, leading to palpitations and an irregular heartbeat.

3. Heat Intolerance: Hyperthyroidism can cause heightened sensitivity to heat, with individuals feeling excessively warm even in normal temperatures.

4. Nervousness and Anxiety: The surplus of thyroid hormones can contribute to heightened nervousness, anxiety, and irritability.

5. Tremors and Muscle Weakness: Fine tremors in the hands and muscle weakness are common manifestations of hyperthyroidism.

6. Excessive Sweating: Increased perspiration, especially during periods of rest, is a common symptom.

7. Changes in Menstrual Patterns: Women with hyperthyroidism may experience irregular menstrual cycles.

Diagnosis involves a combination of clinical evaluation, blood tests to measure thyroid hormone levels, and imaging studies such as thyroid scans. Treatment options aim to restore normal thyroid function and may include antithyroid medications, radioactive iodine therapy, or in severe cases, surgical removal of the thyroid gland.

Effective management of hyperthyroidism requires a collaborative approach involving endocrinologists, primary care physicians, and sometimes, surgeons. Regular monitoring and adjustments to treatment plans are essential to ensure optimal thyroid function and mitigate potential complications associated with an overactive thyroid.

Causes and Symptoms of Hyperthyroidism

Hyperthyroidism, an endocrine disorder, stems from an overactive thyroid gland, leading to the excessive production of thyroid hormones—thyroxine (T4) and triiodothyronine (T3). Understanding the underlying causes and recognizing associated symptoms are critical for the diagnosis and management of this condition.

Causes:

1. Graves' Disease: The most common cause of hyperthyroidism is Graves' disease, an autoimmune disorder. In Graves' disease, the immune system erroneously produces antibodies that stimulate the thyroid gland to produce and release more hormones.

2. Toxic Nodular Goiter: A condition where one or more nodules in the thyroid gland become overactive and produce excess thyroid hormones independently of the body's regulatory mechanisms.

3. Thyroiditis: Inflammation of the thyroid gland, often caused by viral infections, can lead to a temporary release of stored thyroid hormones, resulting in hyperthyroidism.

4. Excessive Iodine Intake: Consuming too much iodine, either through diet or medication, can trigger hyperthyroidism, especially in individuals with underlying thyroid conditions.

5. Tumors: Rarely, tumors of the ovaries or testes (gonadal tumors) or tumors in the pituitary gland can

produce substances that stimulate thyroid hormone production.

Symptoms:

1. Weight Loss: Despite an increased appetite, individuals with hyperthyroidism often experience unintentional weight loss.

2. Increased Heart Rate: Excess thyroid hormones can lead to an elevated heart rate, palpitations, and irregular heartbeat.

3. Heat Intolerance: Individuals may feel overly warm and experience heightened sensitivity to heat.

4. Nervousness and Anxiety: Hyperthyroidism can contribute to increased nervousness, anxiety, and irritability.

5. Tremors and Muscle Weakness: Fine tremors in the hands and muscle weakness are common manifestations of hyperthyroidism.

6. Excessive Sweating: Increased perspiration, even at rest, is a common symptom.

7. Changes in Menstrual Patterns: Women with hyperthyroidism may experience irregular menstrual cycles.

8. Fatigue: Paradoxically, despite the increased metabolic activity, individuals may feel fatigued and weak.

Recognizing these symptoms and seeking medical evaluation is crucial for an accurate diagnosis. Hyperthyroidism, if left untreated, can lead to complications such as heart issues, osteoporosis, and in severe cases, a life-threatening condition known as thyroid storm. Effective management involves addressing the underlying cause and may include medications, radioactive iodine therapy, or surgical intervention to restore thyroid function to normal levels.

Managing the Symptoms of Hyperthyroidism

Hyperthyroidism can present with a range of symptoms, and managing these effectively involves a combination of medical interventions, lifestyle adjustments, and ongoing communication with healthcare professionals. Here's a guide on managing some common symptoms:

1. Fatigue:
  - Balanced Diet: Ensure a well-balanced diet with adequate nutrients, including iron and B vitamins, to combat fatigue.
  - Hydration: Drink plenty of water to stay hydrated, as dehydration can exacerbate fatigue.
  - Rest: Prioritize sufficient rest and quality sleep. Establish a consistent sleep schedule and create a comfortable sleep environment.

2. Increased Heart Rate and Palpitations:
  - Beta-Blockers: Medications like propranolol can help control heart rate and palpitations. Consult with your healthcare provider for appropriate dosages.
  - Stress Reduction Techniques: Practice stress management techniques such as deep breathing, meditation, or yoga to alleviate anxiety and reduce heart rate.

3. Heat Intolerance:
  - Cooling Strategies: Wear lightweight, breathable clothing, and use fans or air conditioning to stay cool.
  - Hydration: Maintain adequate hydration to regulate body temperature.

4. Nervousness and Anxiety:
  - Therapeutic Support: Consider counseling or therapy to address anxiety and provide coping strategies.

- Relaxation Techniques: Practice mindfulness, deep breathing, or progressive muscle relaxation to manage anxiety.

5. Tremors and Muscle Weakness:
- Balanced Nutrition: Consume a diet rich in protein, vitamins, and minerals to support muscle health.
- Moderate Exercise: Engage in moderate exercise, avoiding excessive exertion to prevent muscle weakness.

6. Excessive Sweating:
- Cooling Measures: Wear breathable fabrics and use antiperspirants to manage excessive sweating.
- Hygiene Practices: Maintain good personal hygiene to minimize discomfort.

7. Changes in Weight:
- Nutritional Guidance: Consult with a dietitian to develop a meal plan that supports a healthy weight.
- Regular Monitoring: Regularly monitor weight changes and adjust diet as needed.

General Tips:
- Medication Adherence: Take prescribed medications consistently and attend follow-up appointments to monitor progress.

- Regular Check-ups: Schedule regular check-ups with your healthcare provider for ongoing assessment and adjustment of treatment plans.

- Communication: Communicate openly with your healthcare team about your symptoms, concerns, and any changes you experience.

It's crucial to work closely with healthcare professionals, including endocrinologists and primary care physicians, to tailor a comprehensive treatment plan. Regular monitoring and adjustments to medications or other interventions may be necessary to ensure effective symptom management and overall well-being. Lifestyle modifications can complement medical interventions, promoting a holistic approach to managing hyperthyroidism symptoms.

Drugs Used in Management of Hyperthyroidism

The treatment of hyperthyroidism involves addressing the underlying cause, reducing the production of thyroid hormones, and managing symptoms. The approach may vary based on the severity of symptoms, the cause of hyperthyroidism, and the patient's overall health.

1. Antithyroid Medications:

- *Propylthiouracil (PTU) and Methimazole:* These medications inhibit the production of thyroid hormones by interfering with the activity of the thyroid gland. Methimazole is more commonly prescribed due to its longer duration of action, but PTU may be used in certain situations, such as during the first trimester of pregnancy.

- *Side Effects:* Potential side effects include rash, agranulocytosis (a severe reduction in white blood cell count), liver toxicity (more common with PTU), and, rarely, vasculitis.

2. Beta-Blockers:
- *Propranolol, Atenolol, Metoprolol:* Beta-blockers help manage symptoms such as rapid heart rate, palpitations, and tremors. They do not treat the underlying cause but provide symptomatic relief.

- *Side Effects:* Possible side effects include fatigue, dizziness, and in some cases, exacerbation of underlying lung conditions.

3. Radioactive Iodine Therapy:
- *I-131 Radioactive Iodine:* This treatment aims to destroy thyroid cells, reducing hormone production. It is commonly used for Graves' disease and toxic nodular goiter.

- *Side Effects:* Side effects may include temporary worsening of hyperthyroid symptoms, damage to salivary glands leading to dry mouth, and, rarely, hypothyroidism.

4. Surgery (Thyroidectomy):

- *Partial or Total Thyroidectomy:* Surgical removal of all or part of the thyroid gland is another option, particularly if other treatments are contraindicated or if the goiter is causing compression symptoms.

- *Side Effects:* Potential complications include damage to nearby structures (nerves and parathyroid glands), as well as the risk of hypothyroidism.

Monitoring and Follow-up:
- Regular monitoring of thyroid function tests is crucial to assess the effectiveness of treatment.
- Adjustments to medication dosages may be necessary to maintain thyroid hormone levels within the normal range.

It's essential to discuss the risks, benefits, and potential side effects of each treatment option with a healthcare provider. The choice of treatment depends on factors such as the cause of hyperthyroidism, patient preference, and the presence of other medical conditions. Close collaboration with an endocrinologist ensures a tailored approach to manage hyperthyroidism effectively while minimizing side effects.

Supportive Measures:
Symptomatic Relief: Utilizing medications such as nonsteroidal anti-inflammatory drugs (NSAIDs) for pain relief or anti-anxiety medications for severe anxiety can offer additional comfort.

Monitoring and Follow-Up: Regular monitoring of thyroid function, often through blood tests, is essential to adjust treatment and ensure optimal control of thyroid hormone levels.

Addressing Underlying Causes: If hyperthyroidism is secondary to conditions like toxic nodular goiter or thyroiditis, specific interventions targeting these causes may be necessary.

Patient Education:
Lifestyle Modifications: Encouraging patients to adopt a healthy lifestyle, including stress management, regular exercise, and a well-balanced diet, can contribute to overall well-being.

Adherence to Medication: Educating patients about the importance of adhering to prescribed medications and attending follow-up appointments is crucial for successful management.

CHAPTER SEVEN

Hyothyroidism

Hypothyroidism is a medical condition characterized by an underactive thyroid gland, resulting in insufficient production and release of thyroid hormones—thyroxine (T4) and triiodothyronine (T3). Situated in the neck, the thyroid gland plays a crucial role in regulating metabolism and various physiological functions. In hypothyroidism, the diminished output of thyroid hormones leads to a slowing down of metabolic processes throughout the body.

Common causes of hypothyroidism include autoimmune conditions such as Hashimoto's thyroiditis, where the immune system mistakenly attacks the thyroid tissue, as well as surgical removal of the thyroid gland or radiation therapy. Iodine deficiency, certain medications, and congenital factors can also contribute to hypothyroidism.

Symptoms of hypothyroidism often manifest gradually and may include fatigue, weight gain, cold intolerance, dry skin, brittle hair, and cognitive impairments. Diagnosis involves blood tests measuring thyroid hormone levels, and treatment typically includes lifelong thyroid hormone replacement therapy with medications like levothyroxine to restore hormonal balance. Effective management of hypothyroidism aims to alleviate symptoms, prevent complications, and improve overall well-being. Regular monitoring and adjustments to medication ensure optimal thyroid function.

Causes and Symptoms of Hypothyroidism

Hypothyroidism, a prevalent endocrine disorder, arises from an underactive thyroid gland, leading to diminished production of essential thyroid hormones—thyroxine (T4) and triiodothyronine (T3). Understanding the causes and recognizing associated symptoms are crucial for accurate diagnosis and effective management.

Causes:

1. Autoimmune Thyroiditis (Hashimoto's Disease): The most common cause of hypothyroidism, Hashimoto's disease is an autoimmune condition where the immune

system mistakenly attacks and damages the thyroid tissue, impairing its ability to produce hormones.

2. Surgical Removal of the Thyroid (Thyroidectomy): Individuals who undergo surgical removal of the thyroid gland due to conditions such as thyroid cancer or nodules may develop hypothyroidism.

3. Radiation Therapy: Exposure to therapeutic radiation, particularly around the neck area, can damage thyroid cells and result in hypothyroidism.

4. Iodine Deficiency: In regions with insufficient dietary iodine, the thyroid may struggle to produce an adequate amount of hormones, leading to hypothyroidism.

5. Certain Medications: Some medications, such as lithium (used in psychiatric disorders) and amiodarone (used for heart conditions), can interfere with thyroid function.

6. Congenital Factors: Rarely, individuals may be born with congenital hypothyroidism, where the thyroid gland does not develop properly.

Symptoms:

1. Fatigue: Profound and persistent fatigue is a hallmark symptom of hypothyroidism.

2. Weight Gain: Despite maintaining dietary habits, individuals may experience unexplained weight gain.

3. Cold Intolerance: Sensitivity to cold temperatures and difficulty staying warm are common symptoms.

4. Dry Skin and Hair: Hypothyroidism can lead to dry, flaky skin and brittle hair.

5. Depression and Cognitive Impairment: Mental sluggishness, depression, and difficulty concentrating are cognitive symptoms associated with hypothyroidism.

6. Muscle Weakness and Joint Pain: Weakness in muscles and joints, along with stiffness, may be present.

7. Menstrual Irregularities: Women with hypothyroidism may experience irregularities in their menstrual cycles.

8. Hoarseness: Swelling of the thyroid gland (goiter) can lead to hoarseness or a raspy voice.

Recognizing these symptoms and seeking medical evaluation, particularly when risk factors or family history is present, is essential for timely diagnosis and effective management. Hypothyroidism is typically managed with synthetic thyroid hormone replacement therapy (levothyroxine) to restore normal hormone levels and alleviate symptoms, requiring ongoing monitoring and adjustments to medication dosages.

Management of Hypothyroidism: A Detailed Approach

Effectively managing the symptoms of hypothyroidism involves a comprehensive approach centered on restoring normal thyroid hormone levels, alleviating symptoms, and ensuring optimal well-being. The primary treatment is thyroid hormone replacement therapy, and the most commonly prescribed medication for this purpose is levothyroxine.

Levothyroxine (Synthroid, Levoxyl, Euthyrox):

1. Mechanism of Action: Levothyroxine is a synthetic form of thyroxine (T4), the primary thyroid hormone. It replenishes deficient thyroid hormone levels in the body.

2. Dosage: The prescribed dosage is individualized based on factors such as age, weight, severity of hypothyroidism, and underlying health conditions. It is typically taken orally, preferably in the morning on an empty stomach.

3. Side Effects:
  - Overmedication: Excessive levothyroxine may lead to symptoms of hyperthyroidism, including palpitations, weight loss, and irritability.
  - Allergic Reactions: Some individuals may experience allergic reactions, presenting as rash, itching, or swelling.

4. Monitoring and Adjustments:
  - Regular blood tests, specifically thyroid function tests, are crucial to monitor hormone levels and adjust the dosage as needed.
  - The goal is to achieve and maintain thyroid hormone levels within the normal range.

Supportive Measures:

1. Lifestyle Modifications:
  - Adopting a well-balanced diet rich in essential nutrients, including iodine, is beneficial.
  - Regular exercise can help manage weight and boost overall well-being.

2. Monitoring Symptoms:
  - Regular self-monitoring of symptoms, such as fatigue, weight changes, and mood, aids in assessing the effectiveness of treatment.

3. Patient Education:

- Educating patients on the importance of consistent medication adherence and the need for regular follow-up appointments is crucial.

Potential Complications and Precautions:

1. Cardiovascular Health:
   - Patients with pre-existing cardiovascular conditions may require careful monitoring, as levothyroxine can impact heart rate and blood pressure.

2. Interaction with Other Medications:
   - Levothyroxine may interact with certain medications, such as antacids, calcium supplements, and iron supplements, affecting its absorption. It is advisable to take levothyroxine several hours apart from these medications.

3. Pregnancy:
   - Pregnant women may require adjustments in levothyroxine dosage, as thyroid hormone needs may change during pregnancy.

4. Age Considerations:
   - Dosage adjustments may be necessary in elderly individuals, as they may be more sensitive to the effects of levothyroxine.

Individualized management, regular follow-up, and open communication between healthcare providers and patients are essential components of successful hypothyroidism management. Adjustments to medication dosage, when necessary, aim to optimize thyroid hormone levels and enhance overall quality of life.

CHAPTER EIGHT

Hashimoto's disease

Hashimoto's disease, also known as Hashimoto's thyroiditis, is an autoimmune disorder characterized by chronic inflammation of the thyroid gland. Named after the Japanese physician Dr. Hakaru Hashimoto who first described it in 1912, the condition is the most common cause of hypothyroidism.

In Hashimoto's disease, the immune system mistakenly identifies the thyroid gland's tissues as foreign invaders and produces antibodies that attack and damage the gland. Over time, this autoimmune assault leads to a gradual destruction of thyroid cells, impairing the gland's ability to produce sufficient thyroid hormones—thyroxine (T4) and triiodothyronine (T3).

Hashimoto's disease often progresses slowly, and its early stages may be asymptomatic. As the condition advances, individuals may experience symptoms of hypothyroidism, including fatigue, weight gain, cold intolerance, dry skin, and cognitive difficulties. Diagnosis typically involves blood tests measuring thyroid hormone levels and detecting specific antibodies associated with autoimmune thyroiditis.

Management of Hashimoto's disease often involves thyroid hormone replacement therapy, such as levothyroxine, to address the hormone deficiency and alleviate symptoms. Regular monitoring, lifestyle modifications, and close collaboration with healthcare providers are essential components of effective Hashimoto's disease management.

Exploring the Autoimmune Aspect of Thyroid Disorders

Autoimmune thyroid disorders are a group of conditions where the body's immune system mistakenly targets and attacks the thyroid gland, disrupting its normal function and leading to various thyroid-related disorders. Two primary autoimmune thyroid conditions are Hashimoto's disease and Graves' disease, both characterized by distinct immune system responses.

1. Hashimoto's Disease (Hashimoto's Thyroiditis):

Hashimoto's disease is the most common cause of hypothyroidism, occurring when the immune system produces antibodies that attack the thyroid gland. These antibodies, specifically anti-thyroid peroxidase (TPO) and anti-thyroglobulin (TG) antibodies, gradually damage the thyroid tissue, leading to a decline in thyroid hormone production. As a result, individuals with Hashimoto's disease experience symptoms of hypothyroidism, such as fatigue, weight gain, and cold intolerance.

2. Graves' Disease:

On the other end of the spectrum, Graves' disease is an autoimmune condition causing hyperthyroidism. In Graves' disease, the immune system produces antibodies called thyroid-stimulating immunoglobulins (TSI) that mimic the action of thyroid-stimulating hormone (TSH). These antibodies overstimulate the thyroid gland, leading to an excessive production of thyroid hormones. Individuals with Graves' disease often exhibit symptoms such as weight loss, rapid heart rate, anxiety, and heat intolerance.

Common Themes in Autoimmune Thyroid Disorders:

- Genetic Predisposition: There is often a genetic predisposition to autoimmune thyroid disorders, indicating a hereditary component.

- Environmental Triggers: External factors, such as infections, stress, or hormonal changes, may act as triggers, initiating or exacerbating the autoimmune response against the thyroid.
- Thyroid Antibodies: The presence of specific antibodies, such as anti-TPO and TSI, is a hallmark of autoimmune thyroid disorders and is frequently used in diagnostic testing.

Management:

While autoimmune thyroid disorders are chronic, their symptoms can be effectively managed. Treatment typically involves thyroid hormone replacement therapy for hypothyroidism (as in Hashimoto's disease) or medications, radioactive iodine, or surgery for hyperthyroidism (as in Graves' disease). Balancing thyroid hormone levels and addressing the autoimmune component are key strategies in the comprehensive management of these disorders. Regular monitoring, lifestyle modifications, and a collaborative approach between patients and healthcare providers contribute to optimal outcomes in managing autoimmune thyroid conditions.

Management of Hashimoto's Disease and Graves' Disease: A Comprehensive Approach

Hashimoto's Disease:

1. Levothyroxine (Synthetic Thyroid Hormone):
   - Mechanism of Action: Replaces the deficient thyroid hormones (T4 and T3) to normalize hormone levels.
   - Dosage: Individualized based on blood test results and symptom severity.
   - Side Effects:
     - Overmedication may lead to symptoms of hyperthyroidism.
     - Allergic reactions such as rash or itching are rare.

2. Supportive Measures:
   - Iodine Supplements: If iodine deficiency is a contributing factor.
   - Lifestyle Modifications: A well-balanced diet, stress management, and regular exercise can support overall well-being.

3. Monitoring:
   - Regular Thyroid Function Tests: Periodic blood tests to assess hormone levels and adjust medication dosage.

Graves' Disease:

1. Antithyroid Medications:
   - *Propylthiouracil (PTU) or Methimazole:*
     - Mechanism of Action: Inhibits thyroid hormone production.
     - Dosage: Initially higher, then adjusted based on response.
     - Side Effects:
       - PTU may cause liver complications.
       - Methimazole may cause allergic reactions.

2. Beta-Blockers:
   - *Propranolol, Atenolol, or Metoprolol:*
     - Mechanism of Action: Controls symptoms like rapid heart rate and tremors.
     - Dosage: Adjusted based on symptom severity.
     - Side Effects:
       - Potential for dizziness, fatigue, or low blood pressure.

3. Radioactive Iodine Therapy:
   - *I-131 (Radioiodine):*
     - Mechanism of Action: Destroys thyroid cells to reduce hormone production.
     - Dosage: Administered as a single oral dose.
     - Side Effects:
       - Potential for radiation sickness, transient neck pain, or exacerbation of symptoms before improvement.

4. Surgery (Thyroidectomy):
  - *Partial or Total Thyroid Removal:*
    - Mechanism of Action: Removal of the thyroid gland to eliminate hormone production.
    - Side Effects:
      - Surgical risks, potential for hypothyroidism requiring lifelong hormone replacement.

5. Supportive Measures:
  - *Calcium and Vitamin D Supplements:* Especially if surgery leads to hypoparathyroidism.
    - Regular Monitoring: Assessing thyroid function and addressing any complications promptly.

General Considerations:
- Pregnancy and Breastfeeding: Adjustments to medication dosages and careful monitoring are crucial.
- Side Effect Monitoring: Regularly assess for side effects and adjust treatment accordingly.
- Long-Term Management: Both conditions often require lifelong management and periodic reassessment.

The management of Hashimoto's disease and Graves' disease necessitates a tailored approach, often involving a combination of medications, lifestyle modifications, and, in some cases, definitive interventions like radioactive iodine therapy or surgery. Continuous collaboration between patients and healthcare providers is crucial for effective symptom management, optimizing quality of life, and minimizing potential side effects associated with the chosen treatment modalities. Regular follow-up appointments and ongoing monitoring ensure that treatment plans remain appropriate and adjustments are made as needed.

CHAPTER NINE

Overview of diagnostic tests for

thyroid disorders

Diagnostic tests for thyroid disorders play a crucial role in assessing the health and function of the thyroid gland. These tests help healthcare providers determine whether the thyroid is functioning within normal parameters or if there is an underlying disorder that requires intervention. Here is an overview of key diagnostic tests used in evaluating thyroid disorders:

1. Thyroid Function Tests:
  - TSH (Thyroid-Stimulating Hormone): Elevated TSH levels suggest hypothyroidism, while low levels may indicate hyperthyroidism.

- Free T4 and T3: Measure the levels of active thyroid hormones. Abnormalities can indicate hypo- or hyperthyroidism.

2. Thyroid Antibody Tests:
- Anti-TPO (Thyroid Peroxidase Antibodies) and Anti-Tg (Thyroglobulin Antibodies): Elevated levels indicate autoimmune thyroid disorders like Hashimoto's disease.

3. Radioactive Iodine Uptake (RAIU) Test:
- Measures how much iodine the thyroid absorbs. Helpful in diagnosing hyperthyroidism and determining the cause.

4. Thyroid Imaging:
- Ultrasound: Provides detailed images of the thyroid, helping identify nodules, cysts, or inflammation.
- Thyroid Scan: Involves the use of a radioactive tracer to assess the thyroid's structure and function.

5. Fine Needle Aspiration (FNA) Biopsy:
- Used to evaluate thyroid nodules for the presence of cancerous cells. A thin needle extracts a tissue sample for microscopic examination.

6. Calcitonin Test:
- Measures calcitonin levels, aiding in the diagnosis of medullary thyroid cancer.

7. TRH Stimulation Test:

- Evaluates the pituitary and thyroid response to thyrotropin-releasing hormone (TRH), aiding in the diagnosis of certain thyroid disorders.

8. Thyroid Stimulating Immunoglobulin (TSI) Test:

- Identifies the presence of antibodies associated with Graves' disease.

9. Baseline Metabolic Panel:

- Assesses overall health and may reveal abnormalities associated with thyroid dysfunction.

10. Cholesterol Levels:

- Altered cholesterol levels may be indicative of thyroid dysfunction.

These diagnostic tests are employed based on clinical symptoms, physical examination findings, and the suspected thyroid disorder. Results from these tests help guide healthcare providers in formulating an accurate diagnosis and developing an appropriate treatment plan. Regular monitoring and follow-up testing are essential to track thyroid function over time and ensure effective management of thyroid disorders.

Common medications prescribed for thyroid disorders primarily aim to regulate thyroid hormone levels and manage symptoms associated with either hypothyroidism or hyperthyroidism. Here's an overview of medications commonly used in the treatment of thyroid disorders:

Drugs for Treatment of these Disorders

Hypothyroidism Medications:

1. Levothyroxine (Synthroid, Levoxyl, Euthyrox):
   - Mechanism of Action: Synthetic form of thyroxine (T4), the main thyroid hormone.
   - Dosage: Individualized based on factors like age, weight, and severity of hypothyroidism.
   - Implications: Replaces or supplements the insufficient thyroid hormone, restoring normal levels and alleviating symptoms.

2. Liothyronine (Cytomel):
   - Mechanism of Action: Synthetic form of triiodothyronine (T3), a more active thyroid hormone.
   - Dosage: Used in specific cases where conversion of T4 to T3 is impaired.
   - Implications: Provides a direct source of the active thyroid hormone.

Hyperthyroidism Medications:

1. Thionamides (Methimazole, Propylthiouracil):
   - Mechanism of Action: Inhibit the production of thyroid hormones.
   - Dosage: Adjusted based on thyroid hormone levels.
   - Implications: Effective in managing hyperthyroidism, particularly in Graves' disease.

2. Beta-Blockers (Propranolol, Atenolol, Metoprolol):
   - Mechanism of Action: Controls symptoms like rapid heart rate, tremors, and anxiety by blocking the effects of thyroid hormones.
   - Dosage: Adjusted based on symptom severity.
   - Implications: Provides symptomatic relief while other treatments take effect.

Radioactive Iodine Therapy (I-131):
   - Mechanism of Action: Administered orally, radioactive iodine selectively destroys thyroid cells.
   - Dosage: Single dose determined by the degree of hyperthyroidism.
   - Implications: Often used for long-term management, may lead to hypothyroidism necessitating hormone replacement.

Surgery (Thyroidectomy):
   - Mechanism of Action: Partial or total removal of the thyroid gland.

  - Implications: Resorted to in cases where medications
or radioactive iodine are contraindicated or not well-
tolerated.

Calcitonin:
  - Mechanism of Action: Reduces calcium levels in the
blood.
  - Implications: Used in specific cases like medullary
thyroid cancer.

Considerations and Side Effects:
  - Regular monitoring of thyroid function is crucial to
adjust medication dosages.
  - Side effects may include allergic reactions,
gastrointestinal issues, or complications specific to the
medication used.

Thyroid medications are prescribed based on the specific
diagnosis and individual patient needs. Close
collaboration with healthcare providers ensures the
proper management of thyroid disorders, addressing
symptoms, and optimizing thyroid hormone levels for
overall well-being. Regular follow-up appointments and
monitoring help refine treatment plans and maintain
optimal thyroid function over time.

CHAPTER TEN

A Bridge to Better Health

"A Bridge to Better Health" signifies the journey individuals take to improve their well-being, especially when facing thyroid disorders. This metaphorical bridge connects the challenges of managing thyroid conditions to the destination of improved health and a better quality of life. Here's a reflection on the key elements that construct this bridge:

1. Understanding and Acceptance:
The first step in building a bridge to better health is understanding the nature of thyroid disorders. Whether it's hypothyroidism, hyperthyroidism, or an autoimmune condition like Hashimoto's or Graves' disease, knowledge empowers individuals to make informed decisions about their health. Acceptance of the condition is pivotal, fostering a positive mindset for the journey ahead.

2. Collaboration with Healthcare Providers:

Healthcare professionals serve as architects, guiding individuals across the bridge. Regular communication, adherence to prescribed medications, and participation in recommended therapies are essential. A collaborative approach ensures that the treatment plan is tailored to individual needs and adjusted as necessary.

3. Lifestyle Modifications:

The bridge to better health includes the incorporation of lifestyle changes. This involves adopting a balanced diet, engaging in regular exercise, managing stress, and ensuring adequate sleep. These adjustments contribute not only to the management of thyroid disorders but also to overall well-being.

4. Embracing Holistic Approaches:

Holistic practices form supportive pillars of the bridge. Integrating complementary therapies such as yoga, meditation, and acupuncture can enhance the effectiveness of conventional treatments. These approaches contribute to stress reduction and promote balance in physical and mental health.

5. Education and Advocacy:

Knowledge is a powerful building block. Education about thyroid disorders, treatment options, and potential challenges empowers individuals to advocate for their health. The bridge becomes sturdier as patients actively engage in their care, ask questions, and seek out resources for ongoing learning.

6. Community Support:
The bridge is fortified by a sense of community. Connecting with others facing similar challenges provides a support system. Online forums, support groups, and social networks create spaces for sharing experiences, offering insights, and fostering a sense of camaraderie on the journey to better health.

7. Regular Monitoring and Adjustments:
Continual maintenance ensures the bridge remains strong. Regular check-ups, monitoring thyroid function, and adapting the treatment plan as needed are essential components. This ongoing process allows for adjustments that cater to the dynamic nature of thyroid disorders.

"A Bridge to Better Health" represents a dynamic and personalized journey, acknowledging the challenges while emphasizing the potential for positive transformation. Each step taken, guided by knowledge, collaboration, and a holistic approach, contributes to a stronger bridge, fostering the well-deserved destination of improved health and vitality.

Integrating conventional and alternative therapies is a holistic approach that recognizes the complementary benefits of both medical paradigms, particularly in the management of thyroid disorders. This inclusive strategy harnesses the strengths of conventional medicine and alternative therapies, aiming to provide a comprehensive and personalized path to wellness.

Integrating conventional and alternative therapies

1. Conventional Medicine:

a. Medications:
  - Conventional thyroid medications like levothyroxine or anti-thyroid drugs are often the primary treatment for thyroid disorders. They aim to normalize hormone levels and alleviate symptoms.

b. Radioactive Iodine Therapy and Surgery:
  - In cases of hyperthyroidism or thyroid cancer, conventional treatments like radioactive iodine therapy or thyroidectomy may be recommended.

c. Regular Monitoring:

- Conventional medicine emphasizes regular monitoring through blood tests and imaging, allowing healthcare providers to assess the effectiveness of treatments and make necessary adjustments.

2. Alternative Therapies:

a. Nutritional Approaches:
  - Incorporating dietary changes, including iodine-rich foods and those supporting overall thyroid health, is a common alternative strategy.

b. Herbal Supplements:
  - Herbs like ashwagandha and guggul are believed to have thyroid-supporting properties in alternative medicine.

c. Mind-Body Practices:
  - Techniques such as yoga and meditation, embraced in alternative therapies, contribute to stress reduction, promoting overall well-being.

3. Benefits of Integration:

a. Holistic Wellness:
  - Integrating both conventional and alternative therapies promotes a holistic approach to wellness, addressing physical, mental, and emotional aspects of health.

b. Personalized Care:
   - Tailoring treatment plans to individual needs ensures that patients receive a comprehensive and personalized approach to their healthcare.

c. Enhanced Symptom Management:
   - Alternative therapies can contribute to symptom management, complementing the effects of conventional treatments.

d. Patient Empowerment:
   - Integrative care empowers patients to actively participate in their health journey, making informed decisions about their treatment options.

e. Safety and Efficacy:
   - Integrative care emphasizes safety and efficacy, ensuring that alternative therapies are used judiciously alongside evidence-based conventional treatments.

4. Considerations for Integration:

a. Open Communication:
   - Clear and open communication between patients and healthcare providers is crucial to ensuring seamless integration.

b. Qualified Practitioners:

  - Seek guidance from qualified practitioners, whether in conventional or alternative medicine, to ensure the safety and effectiveness of chosen therapies.

c. Monitoring and Adjustments:
  - Regular monitoring allows for adjustments to the integrated treatment plan based on the individual's response.

In conclusion, the integration of conventional and alternative therapies in the management of thyroid disorders reflects a patient-centered and comprehensive approach. This collaborative strategy, guided by evidence-based practices, empowers individuals to actively engage in their health, fostering a balanced and effective journey toward well-being.

CHAPTER ELEVEN

In-depth exploration of autoimmune aspects in thyroid disorders

An in-depth exploration of the autoimmune aspects in thyroid disorders unveils the intricate interplay between the immune system and the thyroid gland. Autoimmune thyroid disorders, such as Hashimoto's disease and Graves' disease, represent a significant category of thyroid conditions, where the body's immune system mistakenly targets the thyroid tissue, leading to a range of symptoms and complications.

1. Hashimoto's Disease:

Hashimoto's disease is a classic example of an autoimmune thyroid disorder. In this condition, the immune system produces antibodies, specifically anti-thyroid peroxidase (TPO) and anti-thyroglobulin (TG) antibodies, that mistakenly attack the thyroid gland. This chronic inflammation and destruction of thyroid cells lead to hypothyroidism, as the damaged gland becomes less able to produce sufficient thyroid hormones. Individuals with Hashimoto's may experience fatigue, weight gain, and cold intolerance.

2. Graves' Disease:

On the opposite end of the spectrum is Graves' disease, another autoimmune thyroid disorder characterized by hyperthyroidism. In Graves' disease, the immune system produces thyroid-stimulating immunoglobulins (TSI) that mimic the action of thyroid-stimulating hormone (TSH). This results in excessive production of thyroid hormones, causing symptoms such as weight loss, rapid heart rate, and anxiety.

3. Genetic Predisposition:

There is a strong genetic predisposition to autoimmune thyroid disorders, suggesting a hereditary component. Certain gene variations increase the susceptibility to these conditions, and individuals with a family history of autoimmune disorders are at a higher risk.

4. Environmental Triggers:
External factors play a crucial role in triggering autoimmune responses against the thyroid. Infections, stress, and hormonal changes, especially in women postpartum or during menopause, can act as environmental triggers, initiating or exacerbating the autoimmune attack.

5. Role of Thyroid Antibodies:
Measuring thyroid antibodies, such as anti-TPO and TSI, is a key diagnostic tool in identifying autoimmune thyroid disorders. Elevated antibody levels indicate an active autoimmune process, aiding in the confirmation of diagnoses like Hashimoto's or Graves' disease.

6. Implications for Treatment:
Understanding the autoimmune aspects of thyroid disorders is vital for tailoring effective treatment strategies. While conventional treatments like hormone replacement therapy or anti-thyroid medications address symptoms, immune-modulating therapies may be explored in certain cases to target the underlying autoimmune process.

In conclusion, delving into the autoimmune aspects of thyroid disorders sheds light on the intricate mechanisms that drive these conditions. Genetic predisposition, environmental triggers, and the role of specific antibodies contribute to the complexity of autoimmune thyroid disorders. This deeper understanding informs comprehensive treatment approaches aimed at both managing symptoms and modulating the autoimmune response for improved patient outcomes.

Lifestyle changes and therapies for autoimmune conditions

Lifestyle changes and therapies play a significant role in managing autoimmune conditions, including autoimmune thyroid disorders like Hashimoto's disease and Graves' disease. These approaches focus on promoting overall well-being, reducing inflammation, and supporting the immune system. Here's an exploration of lifestyle changes and therapies that can positively impact individuals with autoimmune thyroid disorders:

1. Nutrient-Rich Diet:
A balanced and nutrient-dense diet is foundational for managing autoimmune conditions. Emphasizing foods rich in antioxidants, vitamins, and minerals can help reduce inflammation and support overall health. Incorporating omega-3 fatty acids from sources like fish,

flaxseeds, and walnuts may have anti-inflammatory effects.

2. Gluten-Free Diet:

Some individuals with autoimmune thyroid disorders, particularly Hashimoto's disease, may benefit from a gluten-free diet. Gluten, a protein found in wheat, can potentially trigger an autoimmune response in susceptible individuals. Eliminating or reducing gluten intake may help manage symptoms.

3. Stress Management:

Chronic stress can exacerbate autoimmune conditions. Stress management techniques, such as meditation, yoga, and deep-breathing exercises, play a crucial role in promoting relaxation and reducing the impact of stress on the immune system.

4. Regular Exercise:

Regular physical activity is essential for maintaining a healthy weight, improving mood, and supporting overall well-being. Exercise can also contribute to reducing inflammation and promoting better immune function. However, individuals should choose exercise routines that align with their energy levels and overall health.

5. Sleep Hygiene:

Quality sleep is vital for immune function and overall health. Establishing good sleep hygiene, including maintaining a consistent sleep schedule, creating a conducive sleep environment, and managing stress before bedtime, contributes to better sleep quality.

6. Mind-Body Therapies:
Mind-body therapies, such as acupuncture and biofeedback, focus on the connection between mental and physical well-being. These therapies aim to restore balance within the body and may contribute to symptom management.

7. Functional Medicine and Integrative Care:
Functional medicine approaches focus on addressing the root causes of autoimmune conditions. Integrative care involves collaborating with healthcare providers who specialize in both conventional and complementary approaches to tailor treatment plans to individual needs.

8. Support Groups and Counseling:
Dealing with an autoimmune condition can be emotionally challenging. Joining support groups or seeking counseling provides an avenue for emotional support, coping strategies, and sharing experiences with others facing similar challenges.

9. Environmental Toxin Reduction:
Minimizing exposure to environmental toxins, such as pollutants and certain chemicals, can be beneficial for individuals with autoimmune conditions. This may

involve choosing organic products, avoiding certain household chemicals, and creating a toxin-free living environment.

In conclusion, lifestyle changes and therapies for autoimmune conditions aim to create a supportive environment for the body's natural healing processes. These approaches, when integrated into a comprehensive treatment plan, contribute to managing symptoms, promoting overall well-being, and enhancing the quality of life for individuals with autoimmune thyroid disorders.

CHAPTER TWELVE

Addressing the link between thyroid disorders and vague symptoms

Addressing the link between thyroid disorders and vague symptoms is crucial for accurate diagnosis and effective management. Thyroid disorders, whether hypothyroidism or hyperthyroidism, can manifest with symptoms that may initially appear unrelated or vague, making it challenging to pinpoint the root cause. Recognizing and investigating these vague symptoms is essential for early intervention and improved patient outcomes.

1. Common Vague Symptoms:

Thyroid disorders can present with a range of vague symptoms, including fatigue, weight changes, mood swings, and difficulty concentrating. These symptoms can easily be attributed to various other factors, leading to delayed diagnosis.

2. Comprehensive Evaluation:

Healthcare providers need to conduct a comprehensive evaluation when patients present with vague symptoms. This includes a thorough medical history, physical examination, and consideration of family history, as thyroid disorders often have a genetic component.

3. Thyroid Function Tests:

Testing thyroid function through blood tests measuring thyroid-stimulating hormone (TSH), free thyroxine (T4), and triiodothyronine (T3) levels is a critical step. Abnormalities in these levels can help identify whether the thyroid is overactive (hyperthyroidism) or underactive (hypothyroidism).

4. Consideration of Autoimmune Factors:

Given the autoimmune nature of many thyroid disorders, assessing thyroid antibodies, such as anti-thyroid peroxidase (TPO) and anti-thyroglobulin (TG) antibodies, can provide insights into autoimmune conditions like Hashimoto's disease.

5. Specialist Consultation:

In cases where symptoms persist despite normal thyroid function tests, consultation with an endocrinologist or thyroid specialist may be necessary. Specialized imaging studies, such as thyroid ultrasound, can offer additional information.

6. Individualized Treatment Plans:

Once a thyroid disorder is identified, individualized treatment plans are crucial. For hypothyroidism, synthetic thyroid hormone replacement is commonly prescribed, while hyperthyroidism may involve anti-thyroid medications, radioactive iodine therapy, or surgery.

7. Monitoring and Adjustments:

Regular monitoring of thyroid function is essential to ensure that treatment remains effective. Adjustments to medication dosages may be required to maintain optimal hormone levels and alleviate symptoms.

8. Patient Education:

Educating patients about the link between vague symptoms and thyroid disorders is vital for fostering awareness. Encouraging individuals to seek medical attention for persistent or unexplained symptoms helps in early detection.

9. Holistic Approach:

Considering the holistic aspects of patient health is crucial. Lifestyle modifications, stress management, and addressing any underlying autoimmune components contribute to a comprehensive approach to thyroid disorder management.

In conclusion, addressing the link between thyroid disorders and vague symptoms requires a systematic and thorough approach. Timely recognition, accurate diagnosis, and individualized treatment plans are essential for mitigating the impact of thyroid disorders on overall health and well-being. Healthcare providers play a pivotal role in guiding patients through this process and promoting proactive healthcare seeking for vague symptoms that could indicate an underlying thyroid issue.

Advocating for proper diagnosis and treatment

Advocating for proper diagnosis and treatment of thyroid disorders is essential to ensure optimal health outcomes for individuals facing these conditions. Thyroid disorders, whether hypothyroidism, hyperthyroidism, or autoimmune conditions like Hashimoto's or Graves' disease, often present with a wide range of symptoms that can be misattributed or overlooked. Advocacy in this context involves raising awareness, promoting education, and encouraging proactive healthcare seeking for accurate diagnosis and appropriate treatment.

1. Raising Public Awareness:

Creating awareness about the prevalence and diverse manifestations of thyroid disorders is fundamental to advocacy. Public campaigns, educational materials, and community events can disseminate information about common symptoms, risk factors, and the importance of seeking medical attention for thyroid-related concerns.

2. Empowering Patients:

Empowering individuals to be proactive about their health is a key aspect of advocacy. Educating patients about the signs and symptoms of thyroid disorders, especially those that may be vague or easily dismissed, empowers them to seek timely medical evaluation.

3. Reducing Stigma:

Advocacy plays a role in reducing the stigma associated with thyroid disorders. Some symptoms, such as weight changes or mood swings, may be wrongly attributed to personal habits rather than an underlying medical condition. Normalizing discussions around thyroid health helps eliminate misconceptions and encourages open dialogue.

4. Encouraging Regular Check-ups:

Regular health check-ups and routine screenings are essential components of thyroid advocacy. Encouraging individuals to prioritize preventive care and discussing thyroid function tests with healthcare providers during routine appointments can contribute to early detection.

5. Supporting Comprehensive Testing:

Advocacy involves supporting the importance of comprehensive thyroid testing, including measures of thyroid-stimulating hormone (TSH), free thyroxine (T4), triiodothyronine (T3), and thyroid antibodies. Comprehensive testing is crucial for accurate diagnosis and effective treatment planning.

6. Collaboration with Healthcare Providers:

Advocacy efforts extend to collaboration with healthcare providers. Encouraging healthcare professionals to consider thyroid disorders when evaluating patients with vague or diverse symptoms promotes a more inclusive diagnostic approach.

7. Promoting Patient-Centric Care:

Advocacy emphasizes patient-centric care, where individuals actively participate in decisions about their health. This involves fostering an environment where patients feel heard, respected, and involved in discussions about their symptoms, concerns, and treatment options.

8. Access to Specialist Care:

Ensuring access to specialist care, such as endocrinologists or thyroid specialists, is a vital aspect of advocacy. Timely referrals and consultations with specialists contribute to accurate diagnosis and tailored treatment plans.

9. Addressing Disparities:

Advocacy efforts aim to address healthcare disparities related to thyroid disorders. This involves advocating for equitable access to diagnostic tools, treatments, and education, especially in underserved communities.

In conclusion, advocating for proper diagnosis and treatment of thyroid disorders is a multifaceted effort that involves raising awareness, empowering individuals, and fostering collaboration between patients and healthcare providers. Through these advocacy initiatives, the goal is to enhance early detection, accurate diagnosis, and effective management of thyroid disorders, ultimately improving the overall well-being of individuals impacted by these conditions.

CHAPTER THIRTEEN

The role of inflammation in thyroid

dysfunction

The role of inflammation in thyroid dysfunction is a complex interplay that significantly influences the development and progression of various thyroid disorders. Inflammation is the body's natural response to injury, infection, or perceived threats. In the context of thyroid dysfunction, inflammation can be a contributing factor, particularly in autoimmune thyroid disorders such as Hashimoto's disease and Graves' disease.

1. Autoimmune Thyroid Disorders:
Autoimmune thyroid disorders are characterized by an overactive immune system that mistakenly targets the

thyroid tissue. In Hashimoto's disease, the immune system launches an attack on the thyroid gland, leading to chronic inflammation and gradual destruction of thyroid cells. Conversely, in Graves' disease, the immune system produces antibodies that stimulate the thyroid to overproduce hormones, causing inflammation and hyperthyroidism.

2. Inflammatory Markers:

Elevated levels of inflammatory markers, such as C-reactive protein (CRP) and proinflammatory cytokines, have been observed in individuals with thyroid dysfunction. Chronic inflammation can contribute to the disruption of normal thyroid function and exacerbate symptoms.

3. Impact on Thyroid Hormone Conversion:

Inflammation can interfere with the conversion of inactive thyroid hormone (T4) to its active form (T3) in peripheral tissues. This impaired conversion can contribute to hypothyroidism, as the body may struggle to utilize thyroid hormones effectively.

4. Connection to Thyroid Nodules:

Inflammation has also been linked to the formation of thyroid nodules. Chronic inflammation in the thyroid gland can create a conducive environment for the development of nodules, potentially affecting thyroid function and requiring further evaluation.

5. Environmental Triggers:

Environmental factors, including exposure to pollutants and toxins, can contribute to inflammation in the thyroid gland. Identifying and minimizing exposure to these triggers is essential in managing inflammation and promoting thyroid health.

6. Potential Role in Thyroid Cancer:

In some cases, chronic inflammation may play a role in the development of thyroid cancer. While the exact mechanisms are still under investigation, understanding the inflammatory component is crucial for comprehensive cancer research.

7. Management Strategies:

Addressing inflammation is a key aspect of managing thyroid dysfunction. Lifestyle modifications, including a balanced diet rich in anti-inflammatory foods, stress management techniques, and regular exercise, can help mitigate inflammation.

8. Medications and Anti-Inflammatory Agents:

In certain cases, medications and anti-inflammatory agents may be prescribed to reduce inflammation and manage autoimmune responses. These may include corticosteroids or nonsteroidal anti-inflammatory drugs (NSAIDs), particularly in cases where inflammation is a prominent feature.

9. Holistic Approaches:

Holistic approaches, such as acupuncture and mind-body practices, are increasingly recognized for their potential to reduce inflammation and support overall thyroid health.

Understanding the role of inflammation in thyroid dysfunction is vital for developing targeted interventions and personalized treatment plans. By addressing inflammation, healthcare providers can work towards mitigating its impact on thyroid function and improving the overall well-being of individuals affected by thyroid disorders.

Anti-inflammatory strategies for thyroid health

Anti-inflammatory strategies play a crucial role in promoting thyroid health, particularly in the context of autoimmune thyroid disorders such as Hashimoto's disease and Graves' disease. Chronic inflammation in the thyroid gland can contribute to the progression of these conditions and exacerbate symptoms. Implementing anti-inflammatory approaches is integral to managing inflammation and supporting overall thyroid well-being.

1. Nutrient-Rich Diet:

A diet rich in anti-inflammatory foods can positively impact thyroid health. Incorporating fruits, vegetables, whole grains, and fatty fish with omega-3 fatty acids can help reduce inflammation. Foods like turmeric, ginger, and green tea, known for their anti-inflammatory properties, may also be beneficial.

2. Omega-3 Fatty Acids:

Omega-3 fatty acids, found in fish oil and flaxseeds, have anti-inflammatory effects. Including these sources in the diet can help modulate the inflammatory response and support a healthy balance in the immune system.

3. Gluten-Free Diet:

For individuals with Hashimoto's disease, adopting a gluten-free diet may be recommended. Gluten, found in wheat and related grains, can potentially trigger inflammation and exacerbate autoimmune responses in susceptible individuals.

4. Probiotics:

Gut health is intricately connected to the immune system, and probiotics can contribute to a balanced immune response. Including probiotic-rich foods like yogurt and fermented vegetables can support a healthy gut microbiome and potentially reduce inflammation.

5. Stress Management:

Chronic stress can contribute to inflammation and negatively impact thyroid function. Incorporating stress management techniques such as meditation, deep breathing exercises, and yoga can help mitigate the effects of stress on the immune system.

6. Regular Exercise:
Physical activity is known to have anti-inflammatory effects. Engaging in regular exercise not only supports overall well-being but also helps regulate the immune system and reduce inflammation.

7. Avoiding Environmental Toxins:
Minimizing exposure to environmental toxins and pollutants is crucial for thyroid health. This includes avoiding tobacco smoke, reducing exposure to household chemicals, and choosing organic products when possible.

8. Supplements:
Certain supplements may have anti-inflammatory properties and can be considered under the guidance of a healthcare professional. Vitamin D, selenium, and curcumin supplements, for example, are believed to have anti-inflammatory effects and may support thyroid health.

9. Balanced Lifestyle:

Maintaining a balanced lifestyle that includes adequate sleep, hydration, and regular meals contributes to overall health and supports the body's ability to manage inflammation.

10. Medication Adjustment:
In some cases, medication adjustments may be necessary to address inflammation associated with thyroid disorders. Healthcare providers may consider optimizing thyroid hormone replacement or other specific medications based on individual needs.

Adopting a holistic approach that encompasses anti-inflammatory strategies is essential for managing thyroid disorders effectively. These strategies not only help alleviate symptoms but also contribute to long-term thyroid health and overall well-being. Individuals with thyroid disorders should collaborate with healthcare professionals to tailor these approaches to their specific needs and circumstances.

CHAPTER FOURTEEN

Debunking myths surrounding thyroid function and metabolism

Debunking myths surrounding thyroid function and metabolism is crucial for promoting accurate information and dispelling misconceptions. The thyroid gland plays a central role in regulating metabolism, and misinformation can lead to unnecessary concerns and confusion. Let's explore and debunk some common myths associated with thyroid function and metabolism:

1. Myth: Thyroid Disorders Only Affect Women:
Debunked: While thyroid disorders, especially autoimmune conditions like Hashimoto's and Graves' disease, are more prevalent in women, men can also be affected. Men may experience thyroid dysfunction, and

awareness of symptoms is essential for early diagnosis and management.

2. Myth: Thin People Can't Have Hypothyroidism, and Overweight People Can't Have Hyperthyroidism:
Debunked: Thyroid disorders can affect individuals of any body weight. Hypothyroidism, characterized by an underactive thyroid, can occur in people with various body compositions. Similarly, hyperthyroidism, an overactive thyroid, is not exclusive to individuals who are underweight.

3. Myth: Thyroid Medication Causes Weight Loss or Gain Regardless of Thyroid Levels:
Debunked: Thyroid medication is designed to restore thyroid hormone levels to normal, not induce weight loss or gain directly. Any weight changes associated with thyroid medication are usually related to the correction of thyroid imbalances and not the medication itself.

4. Myth: Everyone with a Slow Metabolism Has Hypothyroidism:
Debunked: Hypothyroidism is one cause of a slow metabolism, but there are various factors influencing metabolism, including age, genetics, and lifestyle. Not everyone with a slow metabolism has thyroid dysfunction.

5. Myth: Thyroid Disorders Only Affect the Metabolism:

Debunked: While thyroid hormones play a crucial role in metabolism, they also impact various body functions, including heart rate, body temperature, and energy levels. Thyroid disorders can affect multiple systems, leading to a range of symptoms beyond metabolic changes.

6. Myth: Thyroid Disorders Are Always Accompanied by Noticeable Symptoms:

Debunked: Thyroid disorders can be asymptomatic or present with subtle symptoms that may be overlooked. Regular thyroid function tests are essential for early detection, especially in individuals at risk due to family history or other factors.

7. Myth: A Single Blood Test Tells Everything About Thyroid Health:

Debunked: Thyroid health is multifaceted, and a comprehensive assessment includes multiple blood tests measuring TSH, free T4, free T3, and thyroid antibodies. A single test may not provide a complete picture of thyroid function.

8. Myth: Dietary Supplements Can Cure Thyroid Disorders:

Debunked: While certain supplements may support overall health, they cannot cure thyroid disorders. Thyroid medication prescribed by healthcare professionals remains the primary treatment for managing thyroid dysfunction.

9. Myth: Thyroid Disorders Are Always Permanent:
Debunked: Some thyroid disorders, especially those of autoimmune origin, may have phases of remission or fluctuations. Individual responses to treatment can vary, and management strategies may need adjustments over time.

Debunking these myths fosters a more accurate understanding of thyroid function and metabolism. It emphasizes the importance of individualized diagnosis, treatment, and ongoing monitoring for those affected by thyroid disorders. Seeking information from reputable sources and consulting healthcare professionals are essential steps in dispelling misconceptions and promoting thyroid health awareness.

Understanding the true impact on metabolism

Understanding the true impact of thyroid function on metabolism reveals the intricate connection between these physiological processes. The thyroid gland, situated in the neck, produces hormones—triiodothyronine (T3) and thyroxine (T4)—that play a pivotal role in regulating metabolism. Metabolism encompasses the body's energy production, utilization, and storage.

Thyroid hormones influence the metabolic rate by affecting the body's utilization of nutrients and oxygen. In cases of hypothyroidism, where the thyroid is underactive, there is a decrease in the production of these hormones, leading to a slower metabolic rate. This can result in symptoms such as fatigue, weight gain, and intolerance to cold temperatures.

Conversely, hyperthyroidism, an overactive thyroid, accelerates the metabolic rate. Excessive production of thyroid hormones prompts increased energy expenditure, causing symptoms such as weight loss, rapid heart rate, and heat intolerance.

The true impact of thyroid function on metabolism extends beyond energy balance; it affects various physiological processes, including cardiovascular function, temperature regulation, and overall cellular activity. Recognizing and managing thyroid-related metabolic changes are crucial for maintaining optimal health and addressing symptoms associated with thyroid dysfunction. Regular monitoring, accurate diagnosis, and tailored treatments are essential components of ensuring a harmonious balance between thyroid function and metabolism.

CHAPTER FIFTEEN

Genetic factors in thyroid disorders

Genetic factors play a significant role in the development of thyroid disorders, contributing to the complex interplay of inherited and environmental influences. Understanding the genetic aspects of thyroid disorders sheds light on their hereditary nature and helps identify individuals at higher risk. Here are key insights into genetic factors in thyroid disorders:

1. Familial Clustering:
Thyroid disorders often exhibit familial clustering, suggesting a genetic predisposition. Individuals with a family history of thyroid disorders, particularly autoimmune conditions like Hashimoto's disease or Graves' disease, are at an increased risk. Shared genetic factors within families contribute to this observed pattern.

2. Heritability Estimates:

Studies indicate a substantial heritability component in thyroid disorders. For instance, in autoimmune thyroid conditions, such as Hashimoto's disease, the heritability estimate is significant, emphasizing the influence of genetic factors in disease susceptibility.

3. Polygenic Inheritance:

Thyroid disorders are generally polygenic, involving the interaction of multiple genes. Certain gene variations contribute to an individual's susceptibility to thyroid dysfunction. The Human Leukocyte Antigen (HLA) complex, among other genetic loci, has been implicated in autoimmune thyroid disorders.

4. Shared Genetic Links:

Genetic factors may contribute to the co-occurrence of different thyroid disorders within families. For example, a shared genetic susceptibility might contribute to the occurrence of both hyperthyroidism and hypothyroidism in different family members.

5. Specific Gene Associations:

Specific genes have been identified as associated with thyroid disorders. For instance, variations in the TPO (thyroid peroxidase) and Tg (thyroglobulin) genes are linked to autoimmune thyroid diseases. Understanding these specific gene associations enhances the understanding of the underlying mechanisms of thyroid dysfunction.

6. Environmental Triggers and Gene Interactions:
While genetic factors are crucial, environmental triggers play a role in the development of thyroid disorders. Interactions between genetic susceptibility and environmental factors, such as infections, stress, and iodine exposure, contribute to the manifestation of thyroid dysfunction.

7. Advances in Genetic Research:
Advancements in genetic research, including genome-wide association studies (GWAS), have facilitated the identification of novel genetic markers associated with thyroid disorders. These studies enhance our understanding of the genetic landscape and potential therapeutic targets.

8. Implications for Personalized Medicine:
Recognizing the genetic underpinnings of thyroid disorders holds promise for personalized medicine. Genetic information can inform risk assessments, guide early interventions, and contribute to tailored treatment approaches based on an individual's genetic profile.

In conclusion, genetic factors significantly influence the susceptibility and development of thyroid disorders. A nuanced understanding of the genetic landscape enhances our ability to identify at-risk individuals, predict disease outcomes, and advance personalized approaches to managing thyroid dysfunction. Integrating genetic information into clinical practice holds potential for more targeted and effective interventions in the realm of thyroid health.

Balancing genetic predisposition with lifestyle choices

Balancing genetic predisposition with lifestyle choices is a dynamic approach to mitigating the impact of genetic factors on health outcomes, particularly in the context of conditions like thyroid disorders. While genetics play a crucial role in determining susceptibility to certain conditions, lifestyle choices can modulate gene expression and influence overall well-being. Here's a closer look at how individuals can navigate the interplay between genetic predisposition and lifestyle for optimal health:

1. Lifestyle Modifications:
Adopting a healthy lifestyle can help offset genetic predispositions. Regular exercise, a balanced diet rich in nutrients, and adequate sleep contribute to overall well-being. In the context of thyroid disorders, these lifestyle modifications can positively influence metabolism, immune function, and stress management.

2. Nutritional Choices:

Nutritional choices are pivotal in managing genetic predispositions. For individuals with a family history of thyroid disorders, paying attention to iodine intake, incorporating selenium-rich foods, and considering a balanced, anti-inflammatory diet may be beneficial. Tailoring nutritional choices to individual needs can help support thyroid health.

3. Stress Management:

Genetic predisposition can contribute to stress susceptibility, and chronic stress is known to impact overall health, including thyroid function. Adopting stress management techniques such as mindfulness, meditation, or yoga can help modulate the physiological response to stressors.

4. Environmental Factors:

Environmental factors, including exposure to pollutants and toxins, can interact with genetic predispositions. Making conscious choices to minimize exposure, such as using eco-friendly products and avoiding tobacco smoke, contributes to a healthier environment for individuals with genetic susceptibilities.

5. Regular Health Check-ups:

Individuals with a genetic predisposition to thyroid disorders should prioritize regular health check-ups.

Monitoring thyroid function through routine blood tests allows for early detection and intervention, helping to manage potential health challenges proactively.

6. Personalized Medicine:

Advances in genetic research have paved the way for personalized medicine. Understanding one's genetic predisposition can inform healthcare decisions, allowing for tailored interventions and treatments that consider individual genetic variations.

7. Collaboration with Healthcare Providers:

Open communication and collaboration with healthcare providers are crucial. Individuals should share their family medical history and work with healthcare professionals to create personalized health plans that align with both genetic factors and lifestyle choices.

8. Holistic Wellness Approach:

A holistic wellness approach considers the interconnectedness of various lifestyle factors. Balancing nutrition, physical activity, stress management, and adequate sleep forms a comprehensive strategy to support overall health and mitigate the impact of genetic predispositions.

In conclusion, while genetic predispositions may set the stage for certain health outcomes, lifestyle choices play a pivotal role in shaping health trajectories. Individuals have the power to influence their well-being through mindful lifestyle decisions that complement their genetic makeup. Balancing genetic predisposition with proactive and health-conscious choices empowers individuals to take charge of their health and work towards optimal well-being.

CHAPTER SIXTEEN

Exploring the role of lifestyle in

thyroid health

Exploring the role of lifestyle in thyroid health is integral to understanding how daily habits and choices significantly impact the function of the thyroid gland. The thyroid, a small but mighty gland located in the neck, plays a crucial role in regulating metabolism, energy production, and overall well-being. Here's a detailed exploration of the key lifestyle factors that influence thyroid health:

1. Nutrition:

A balanced and nutrient-rich diet is fundamental to supporting thyroid function. Essential nutrients like iodine, selenium, zinc, and vitamins such as B and D play critical roles in thyroid hormone synthesis and conversion. Including a variety of whole foods, such as fruits, vegetables, lean proteins, and whole grains, contributes to optimal thyroid health.

2. Iodine Intake:

Iodine is a key component in thyroid hormone production. While iodine is essential, excessive or inadequate intake can disrupt thyroid function. Striking a balance by incorporating iodine-rich foods like seaweed and iodized salt can help maintain optimal iodine levels.

3. Stress Management:

Chronic stress can adversely affect the thyroid gland and hormone levels. The stress hormone cortisol, when elevated over prolonged periods, may interfere with thyroid function. Incorporating stress management techniques such as meditation, yoga, and deep-breathing exercises supports overall well-being and thyroid health.

4. Physical Activity:

Regular exercise is beneficial for metabolism and overall health. Physical activity can help regulate thyroid hormone levels and contribute to weight management. Finding a balance in the intensity and type of exercise that aligns with individual preferences and health status is key.

5. Adequate Sleep:

Quality sleep is essential for thyroid health and overall well-being. During sleep, the body undergoes repair and restoration processes, including the regulation of hormones. Establishing good sleep hygiene and ensuring sufficient rest contributes to a healthy thyroid.

6. Avoiding Environmental Toxins:

Exposure to environmental toxins and pollutants can impact thyroid function. Minimizing exposure by choosing organic products, reducing reliance on plastics, and avoiding tobacco smoke contributes to a healthier environment for the thyroid.

7. Balancing Hormones:

Hormonal balance is interconnected with thyroid health. Women, in particular, may experience fluctuations in thyroid function during hormonal changes, such as pregnancy or menopause. Managing hormonal health through regular check-ups and lifestyle choices supports thyroid function.

8. Regular Check-ups:

Routine health check-ups, including thyroid function tests, are essential for early detection of potential issues. Regular monitoring allows for timely intervention and management, promoting optimal thyroid health.

9. Individualized Approaches:

Recognizing that lifestyle needs vary among individuals, adopting an individualized approach to lifestyle choices is crucial. Tailoring nutrition, exercise, and stress management strategies to align with personal preferences and health goals contributes to sustainable changes.

In conclusion, lifestyle choices play a pivotal role in maintaining and promoting thyroid health. By adopting a holistic approach that encompasses nutrition, stress management, physical activity, and environmental awareness, individuals can positively influence their thyroid function and overall well-being. Consulting with healthcare professionals for personalized guidance ensures that lifestyle choices align with individual health needs and goals.

Empowering readers to take control of their well-being

Empowering readers to take control of their well-being is a transformative journey that involves providing knowledge, fostering self-awareness, and encouraging proactive choices for a healthier and more fulfilling life. Here's a comprehensive exploration of how readers can take charge of their well-being:

1. Knowledge is Key:

Empowerment begins with knowledge. Providing readers with accurate, accessible, and comprehensible information about various aspects of health, including nutrition, exercise, mental well-being, and disease prevention, equips them to make informed decisions about their lifestyle and healthcare.

2. Encouraging Self-Awareness:

Encouraging readers to cultivate self-awareness is crucial. This involves understanding one's body, recognizing individual needs and preferences, and being attuned to the impact of lifestyle choices on physical and mental health. Mindfulness practices, journaling, and reflective exercises can aid in developing self-awareness.

3. Setting Realistic Goals:

Empowerment involves setting realistic and achievable health goals. Breaking down larger objectives into manageable steps makes the journey more attainable. Whether it's incorporating regular exercise, improving dietary habits, or managing stress, setting specific, measurable, and realistic goals promotes sustained well-being.

4. Building Healthy Habits:

Encouraging the establishment of healthy habits is fundamental to taking control of well-being. Consistent engagement in activities that promote physical, mental, and emotional health, such as regular exercise, balanced nutrition, and sufficient sleep, contributes to a holistic and sustainable approach to well-being.

5. Stress Management Techniques:

Equipping readers with stress management techniques is essential in today's fast-paced world. Techniques like meditation, deep breathing, and mindfulness can help individuals navigate stressors, promoting mental resilience and overall well-being.

6. Regular Health Check-ups:

Empowering readers involves emphasizing the importance of regular health check-ups. Routine screenings, preventive healthcare measures, and staying informed about individual health metrics contribute to early detection and proactive management of potential health issues.

7. Embracing a Holistic Approach:

Taking control of well-being requires embracing a holistic approach that considers physical, mental, and emotional aspects. Encouraging readers to address their overall health, rather than focusing on isolated components, fosters a comprehensive understanding of well-being.

8. Seeking Professional Guidance:

Empowerment involves recognizing when professional guidance is needed. Encouraging readers to consult healthcare professionals, nutritionists, and mental health experts ensures that their well-being journey is guided by evidence-based practices and personalized advice.

9. Cultivating a Supportive Environment:
A supportive environment is crucial for well-being. Encouraging readers to foster positive relationships, seek support from friends and family, and engage in communities that promote health-conscious lifestyles enhances the well-being journey.

10. Celebrating Progress:
Empowerment also involves celebrating small victories and progress. Acknowledging achievements, no matter how modest, reinforces positive behaviors and motivates individuals to continue their well-being journey.

In conclusion, empowering readers to take control of their well-being is a multifaceted endeavor that encompasses education, self-awareness, goal-setting, and holistic approaches. By providing the tools and knowledge needed for informed decision-making, individuals can embark on a journey toward a healthier, more empowered, and fulfilling life.

Strategies for rebuilding and supporting thyroid health involve a multifaceted approach that addresses various aspects of lifestyle, nutrition, and overall well-being. Whether dealing with thyroid disorders, such as hypothyroidism or autoimmune conditions like Hashimoto's or Graves' disease, adopting these strategies can contribute to improved thyroid function and overall health.

CHAPTER SEVENTEEN

Strategies for rebuilding and

supporting thyroid health

1. Optimal Nutrition:
Ensuring proper nutrition is vital for supporting thyroid health. Incorporating foods rich in iodine, selenium, zinc, and vitamins such as B and D can support thyroid hormone production. A balanced diet with a variety of nutrient-dense foods promotes overall well-being.

2. Iodine Balance:
Maintaining a balance in iodine intake is crucial, especially for individuals with thyroid disorders. While iodine is essential for thyroid function, excessive intake can be detrimental. Consulting with a healthcare

professional or nutritionist to determine appropriate iodine levels is advisable.

3. Thyroid-Supporting Supplements:
Supplements like selenium, zinc, and omega-3 fatty acids have been associated with supporting thyroid health. However, supplementation should be done under the guidance of a healthcare professional to ensure appropriate dosages and prevent interactions with medications.

4. Stress Management:
Chronic stress can adversely affect thyroid function. Incorporating stress management techniques, such as meditation, yoga, and deep-breathing exercises, helps modulate the body's stress response and supports overall thyroid health.

5. Regular Exercise:
Physical activity contributes to metabolic regulation and overall well-being. Regular exercise, tailored to individual fitness levels, promotes optimal thyroid function and helps manage weight, a common concern in thyroid disorders.

6. Adequate Sleep:
Quality sleep is essential for thyroid health and overall hormonal balance. Establishing consistent sleep patterns

and creating a conducive sleep environment supports the body's repair and restoration processes.

7. Limiting Environmental Toxins:
Minimizing exposure to environmental toxins and pollutants is beneficial for thyroid health. Choosing organic products, reducing the use of plastics, and avoiding tobacco smoke contribute to a healthier environment.

8. Regular Health Monitoring:
Individuals with thyroid disorders should undergo regular health check-ups to monitor thyroid hormone levels and overall health. Routine screenings allow for early detection of any changes that may require adjustments in treatment or lifestyle.

9. Mindful Practices:
Incorporating mindful practices, such as meditation and deep-breathing exercises, supports both mental and physical well-being. Mindfulness can help manage stress, improve focus, and positively impact overall health.

10. Consultation with Healthcare Professionals:
Working closely with healthcare professionals, including endocrinologists and nutritionists, is crucial. Tailoring strategies to individual needs and regularly reviewing progress ensures a personalized and effective approach to rebuilding and supporting thyroid health.

In conclusion, rebuilding and supporting thyroid health involve a holistic approach that considers nutrition, lifestyle, and overall well-being. By incorporating these strategies and collaborating with healthcare professionals, individuals can optimize their thyroid function and enhance their quality of life.

Lifestyle changes for long-term well-being

Adopting lifestyle changes for long-term well-being is a proactive and sustainable approach to achieving and maintaining optimal health. These changes encompass various aspects of daily life, promoting physical, mental, and emotional well-being. Here's a comprehensive exploration of key lifestyle changes that contribute to long-term health:

1. Balanced Nutrition:
A cornerstone of long-term well-being is a balanced and nutritious diet. Prioritizing whole foods, including fruits, vegetables, lean proteins, and whole grains, provides essential nutrients for overall health. Maintaining a balanced diet supports energy levels, immune function, and disease prevention.

2. Regular Physical Activity:

Incorporating regular exercise into daily routines is vital for long-term well-being. Physical activity contributes to cardiovascular health, weight management, and overall fitness. Finding activities that bring joy and suit individual preferences ensures sustainable engagement over time.

3. Adequate Sleep:

Quality sleep is essential for physical and mental health. Establishing consistent sleep patterns, creating a comfortable sleep environment, and prioritizing sufficient rest contribute to improved cognitive function, emotional well-being, and overall vitality.

4. Stress Management Techniques:

Chronic stress can have detrimental effects on health. Adopting stress management techniques, such as meditation, mindfulness, or yoga, helps mitigate the impact of stressors and fosters emotional resilience.

5. Hydration:

Maintaining proper hydration is often underestimated but is crucial for various bodily functions. Drinking an adequate amount of water supports digestion, nutrient absorption, and overall cellular function.

6. Limiting Alcohol and Tobacco:

Reducing or eliminating alcohol consumption and avoiding tobacco products are significant lifestyle changes for long-term well-being. Both substances can have detrimental effects on physical health and increase the risk of various diseases.

7. Regular Health Check-ups:

Proactive health monitoring through regular check-ups is essential for preventive care. Routine screenings and consultations with healthcare professionals allow for early detection of potential health issues, enabling timely intervention.

8. Mindfulness and Mental Health Practices:

Cultivating mental well-being through mindfulness practices, therapy, or engaging in hobbies promotes emotional resilience. Focusing on mental health is a crucial aspect of long-term well-being.

9. Social Connections:

Maintaining meaningful social connections contributes to overall well-being. Building and nurturing relationships provide emotional support, reduce feelings of isolation, and contribute to a sense of community.

10. Continual Learning and Personal Growth:

Engaging in continual learning and personal growth fosters a sense of purpose and fulfillment. Pursuing hobbies, acquiring new skills, and setting goals contribute to a positive outlook on life and long-term satisfaction.

11. Environmental Awareness:

Being mindful of environmental impact and making sustainable choices supports both personal and planetary well-being. Reducing waste, choosing eco-friendly products, and appreciating nature contribute to long-term health.

12. Positive Mindset:

Adopting a positive mindset is foundational for long-term well-being. Cultivating gratitude, practicing optimism, and reframing challenges as opportunities for growth contribute to a resilient and positive outlook on life.

In conclusion, embracing these lifestyle changes fosters a holistic and enduring approach to well-being. By incorporating these habits into daily life and adapting them to individual preferences and needs, individuals can embark on a lifelong journey towards sustained health and happiness.

CHAPTER EIGHTEEN

Life Without Thyroid

Coping with a thyroidectomy, the surgical removal of the thyroid gland, and adjusting to life without a thyroid is a significant transition that requires both physical and emotional adaptation. The thyroid plays a crucial role in regulating metabolism, energy levels, and overall well-being, so its absence necessitates careful management to maintain a healthy and balanced life.

1. Hormone Replacement Therapy:
Following a thyroidectomy, individuals typically require lifelong hormone replacement therapy. Thyroid hormone medications, such as levothyroxine, are prescribed to replace the hormones that the thyroid would naturally produce. Regular monitoring and adjustments in medication dosage are crucial to maintain optimal hormone levels.

2. Emotional Support:

The emotional impact of living without a thyroid can be profound. Some individuals may experience feelings of loss, anxiety, or uncertainty about managing their health. Seeking emotional support from friends, family, or support groups can be beneficial in navigating these challenges.

3. Lifestyle Modifications:

Adapting to life without a thyroid often involves making lifestyle modifications. Paying close attention to nutrition, stress management, and regular exercise becomes essential to support overall well-being and help manage potential weight changes.

4. Dietary Considerations:

Certain dietary considerations are important for those without a thyroid. Maintaining consistent iodine levels, not exceeding recommended limits, and being mindful of nutrient intake, especially calcium and vitamin D, contribute to overall health.

5. Regular Medical Check-ups:

Continual monitoring of thyroid hormone levels and overall health through regular medical check-ups is crucial. This allows healthcare professionals to assess the effectiveness of hormone replacement therapy, address any complications, and provide ongoing guidance.

6. Managing Symptoms:

Individuals may experience symptoms related to thyroid hormone imbalances, such as fatigue, weight changes, and mood swings. Identifying and managing these symptoms promptly, in collaboration with healthcare providers, ensures a better quality of life.

7. Patient Education:

Educating oneself about the intricacies of living without a thyroid is empowering. Understanding the role of thyroid hormones, the importance of medication adherence, and potential lifestyle adjustments contributes to effective self-management.

8. Supportive Healthcare Team:

Building a supportive healthcare team is critical. Working closely with endocrinologists, surgeons, and other specialists ensures comprehensive and individualized care. Regular communication with healthcare providers facilitates proactive management of thyroid-related concerns.

9. Adjusting to Medication Routines:

Incorporating thyroid hormone medication into daily routines is a lifelong commitment. Establishing consistent medication habits, such as taking medications on an empty stomach and avoiding interactions with other medications or supplements, is crucial for optimal effectiveness.

10. Wellness Practices:

Engaging in wellness practices, such as mindfulness, relaxation techniques, and stress-reducing activities, contributes to overall health. These practices support emotional well-being and help individuals cope with the adjustments associated with life without a thyroid.

In conclusion, coping with a thyroidectomy and adapting to life without a thyroid involves a holistic and individualized approach. Through a combination of medical management, emotional support, and lifestyle adjustments, individuals can successfully navigate this transition and lead fulfilling lives. Regular communication with healthcare professionals and ongoing self-care practices are key components of effectively managing life without a thyroid.

Managing hormonal balance through medication

Managing hormonal balance through medication is a critical aspect of addressing various health conditions where hormone levels play a pivotal role. Hormones act as messengers in the body, influencing processes such as metabolism, growth, mood, and reproductive functions. When hormonal imbalances occur, medications are often prescribed to restore equilibrium. Here's an exploration of how medications are utilized to manage hormonal balance:

1. Hormone Replacement Therapy (HRT):
In conditions where the body's natural hormone production is insufficient, Hormone Replacement Therapy (HRT) is commonly employed. For instance, women experiencing menopausal symptoms may be prescribed estrogen and progesterone to alleviate symptoms like hot flashes, mood swings, and sleep disturbances.

2. Thyroid Hormone Medications:
Thyroid disorders, such as hypothyroidism or hyperthyroidism, often require medication to regulate thyroid hormone levels. Levothyroxine is a common medication prescribed to replace or supplement thyroid hormones for individuals with an underactive thyroid.

3. Insulin and Diabetes Medications:
For individuals with diabetes, maintaining insulin balance is crucial. Medications such as insulin injections or oral hypoglycemic agents help regulate blood sugar levels, promoting optimal glucose metabolism.

4. Birth Control Pills:

Oral contraceptives are widely used to regulate hormonal fluctuations in women. By controlling estrogen and progesterone levels, birth control pills prevent ovulation and provide various benefits, including contraception, menstrual cycle regulation, and acne control.

5. Corticosteroids:

Corticosteroids are prescribed to manage conditions related to adrenal hormone imbalances. These medications, such as prednisone, can suppress inflammation and modulate the immune response in conditions like autoimmune disorders or adrenal insufficiency.

6. Anti-androgen Medications:

In conditions characterized by excessive androgen production, such as polycystic ovary syndrome (PCOS), anti-androgen medications may be prescribed to reduce the effects of male hormones. These medications can help manage symptoms like acne and hirsutism.

7. Selective Estrogen Receptor Modulators (SERMs):

SERMs are medications that selectively modulate estrogen receptors in the body. They are used in conditions like breast cancer prevention or treatment, as well as in osteoporosis management, where maintaining hormonal balance is crucial.

8. Gonadotropin-Releasing Hormone (GnRH) Agonists/Antagonists:

In reproductive health, medications that affect the secretion of gonadotropin-releasing hormone (GnRH) are utilized. These medications play a role in managing conditions like endometriosis, uterine fibroids, and certain fertility treatments.

9. Anti-thyroid Medications:

For individuals with hyperthyroidism, anti-thyroid medications like methimazole or propylthiouracil may be prescribed to reduce the production of excess thyroid hormones and restore hormonal balance.

10. Osteoporosis Medications:

In postmenopausal women or individuals at risk of osteoporosis, medications such as bisphosphonates or hormone therapies may be prescribed to maintain bone density and hormonal balance.

11. Testosterone Replacement Therapy (TRT):

In conditions where testosterone levels are deficient, such as hypogonadism, Testosterone Replacement Therapy (TRT) may be recommended. This therapy helps restore normal testosterone levels and address associated symptoms.

12. Monitoring and Adjustments:

Managing hormonal balance through medication involves regular monitoring of hormone levels and adjusting medication dosages as needed. This dynamic process ensures that hormonal equilibrium is maintained over time.

In conclusion, medications play a pivotal role in managing hormonal imbalances and restoring equilibrium in the body. Healthcare professionals carefully consider individual needs and conditions, prescribing medications tailored to address specific hormonal challenges. Regular monitoring, adherence to medication regimens, and collaboration with healthcare providers are essential components of successful hormonal balance management through medication.

CHAPTER NINETEEN

Nutritional approaches to support thyroid health

Nutritional approaches play a crucial role in supporting thyroid health, as the thyroid gland relies on specific nutrients for the synthesis and regulation of thyroid hormones. A well-balanced and nutrient-dense diet can contribute to optimal thyroid function. Here's an exploration of key nutritional approaches to support thyroid health:

1. Iodine-Rich Foods:
Iodine is a vital component of thyroid hormones, and its deficiency can lead to thyroid dysfunction. Including iodine-rich foods in the diet, such as seaweed, fish, dairy

products, and iodized salt in moderation, helps maintain optimal iodine levels.

2. Selenium Sources:
Selenium is essential for the conversion of thyroid hormones. Incorporating selenium-rich foods like Brazil nuts, sunflower seeds, fish, and eggs supports the production and utilization of thyroid hormones.

3. Zinc Inclusion:
Zinc plays a role in thyroid hormone regulation and immune function. Foods like meat, shellfish, nuts, seeds, and dairy products are good sources of zinc. Ensuring an adequate intake of zinc supports overall thyroid health.

4. Omega-3 Fatty Acids:
Omega-3 fatty acids have anti-inflammatory properties and may help reduce inflammation associated with certain thyroid disorders. Fatty fish, flaxseeds, chia seeds, and walnuts are excellent sources of omega-3 fatty acids.

5. Balanced Macronutrients:
Maintaining a well-balanced ratio of macronutrients—carbohydrates, proteins, and fats—is essential for overall health, including thyroid function. A balanced diet ensures a steady supply of energy and nutrients needed for various physiological processes.

6. Vitamins A and D:

Vitamins A and D are crucial for thyroid hormone synthesis and function. Foods rich in vitamin A include sweet potatoes, carrots, and leafy greens, while vitamin D sources include fatty fish, egg yolks, and fortified dairy products.

7. Fiber-Rich Foods:
Adequate fiber intake supports digestive health and may assist in preventing constipation, a common symptom in hypothyroidism. Whole grains, fruits, vegetables, and legumes are excellent sources of fiber.

8. Goitrogenic Foods in Moderation:
Some foods contain goitrogens, compounds that can interfere with thyroid function when consumed in excess. Cooking these foods can reduce goitrogenic effects. Examples include cruciferous vegetables like broccoli, cabbage, and Brussels sprouts.

9. Hydration:
Staying well-hydrated is essential for overall health, including thyroid function. Water supports the transport of hormones and nutrients throughout the body, ensuring optimal cellular function.

10. Limiting Processed Foods and Sugar:
Reducing the intake of processed foods and added sugars supports overall health and helps maintain a

stable blood sugar level. Imbalances in blood sugar can impact hormonal regulation, including thyroid function.

11. Gluten Sensitivity Awareness:

In some cases, individuals with autoimmune thyroid conditions, such as Hashimoto's disease, may benefit from being aware of gluten sensitivity. Some people find that reducing or eliminating gluten from their diet helps manage autoimmune-related symptoms.

12. Consultation with a Healthcare Professional:

Individual nutritional needs can vary, and consulting with a healthcare professional or a registered dietitian ensures personalized guidance. They can provide recommendations based on individual health conditions, medication interactions, and specific dietary preferences.

In conclusion, adopting a well-rounded and nutrient-dense diet is fundamental for supporting thyroid health. By incorporating these nutritional approaches into daily habits, individuals can positively impact thyroid function and contribute to overall well-being. It's important to approach dietary changes with awareness of individual needs and consult with healthcare professionals for personalized guidance.

Integrating herbs and supplements into a balanced diet

Integrating herbs and supplements into a balanced diet can be a complementary approach to support overall health and well-being. While a balanced diet provides essential nutrients, herbs and supplements may offer additional benefits in promoting specific health goals or addressing individual needs. Here's an exploration of how to integrate these elements effectively:

1. Herbal Teas:
Incorporating herbal teas into daily routines is a simple way to enjoy the benefits of herbs. For example, chamomile tea may promote relaxation and aid in digestion, while peppermint tea can have soothing effects on the digestive system.

2. Adaptogenic Herbs:
Adaptogenic herbs, such as ashwagandha and rhodiola, are known for their ability to help the body adapt to stress. These herbs may be taken in supplement form or added to smoothies and recipes for a convenient integration into the diet.

3. Turmeric and Curcumin:

Turmeric, with its active compound curcumin, is celebrated for its anti-inflammatory properties. Including turmeric in cooking or taking curcumin supplements can contribute to overall well-being.

4. Omega-3 Supplements:
While fatty fish, flaxseeds, and walnuts are natural sources of omega-3 fatty acids, supplements can provide additional support for cardiovascular health and cognitive function. Fish oil or algae-based omega-3 supplements are common choices.

5. Vitamin D Supplementation:
Vitamin D is crucial for bone health and immune function. For individuals with limited sun exposure, vitamin D supplements may be recommended, especially during seasons with less sunlight.

6. Probiotics:
Probiotic supplements or fermented foods like yogurt, kefir, and sauerkraut contribute to gut health. They contain beneficial bacteria that support digestion and immune function.

7. Ginseng and Ginkgo Biloba:
Ginseng is believed to enhance energy and vitality, while ginkgo biloba may support cognitive function. These herbs can be taken in supplement form or integrated into teas and recipes.

8. Magnesium Supplements:

Magnesium is essential for various bodily functions, including muscle and nerve function. Magnesium supplements or magnesium-rich foods like leafy greens and nuts can be included in the diet.

9. Herbal Supplements for Sleep:

Herbs such as valerian root and passionflower are known for their calming effects and may be used in supplement form to promote better sleep.

10. Consultation with a Healthcare Professional:

Before integrating herbs and supplements into a diet, it's important to consult with a healthcare professional. They can provide guidance based on individual health needs, potential interactions with medications, and appropriate dosages.

11. Consider Whole Foods First:

While supplements can be beneficial, obtaining nutrients from whole foods is generally preferable. A balanced diet rich in fruits, vegetables, whole grains, and lean proteins should form the foundation of a healthy lifestyle.

12. Personalized Approach:

Each person's nutritional needs are unique. Tailoring the integration of herbs and supplements to individual health goals and concerns ensures a personalized and effective approach.

In conclusion, integrating herbs and supplements into a balanced diet can enhance overall health and address specific wellness goals. However, it's crucial to approach supplementation mindfully, considering individual needs, consulting with healthcare professionals, and prioritizing whole foods as the primary source of nutrients.

CHAPTER TWENTY

Rehabilitation exercises and practices for thyroid health

Rehabilitation exercises and practices can be valuable components of a comprehensive approach to supporting thyroid health. While exercise alone cannot cure thyroid disorders, it can contribute to overall well-being, help manage symptoms, and enhance the effectiveness of medical treatments. Here's an exploration of rehabilitation exercises and practices beneficial for thyroid health:

1. Aerobic Exercise:
Regular aerobic exercise, such as brisk walking, jogging, cycling, or swimming, can promote cardiovascular health and assist in weight management. For individuals with

thyroid disorders, maintaining a healthy weight is important, as excessive weight can exacerbate symptoms.

2. Strength Training:
Incorporating strength training exercises, such as weightlifting or bodyweight exercises, helps build muscle mass. This is particularly beneficial for individuals with hypothyroidism, as it can counteract muscle weakness and fatigue associated with the condition.

3. Yoga:
Yoga is known for its stress-reducing benefits and may help manage symptoms related to thyroid disorders. Specific yoga poses, such as shoulder stands and fish pose, are believed to stimulate the thyroid gland and improve overall thyroid function.

4. Tai Chi:
Tai Chi, an ancient Chinese martial art, combines slow, flowing movements with deep breathing. This low-impact exercise can improve balance, flexibility, and mental well-being, making it suitable for individuals with varying fitness levels, including those with thyroid conditions.

5. Pilates:
Pilates focuses on core strength, flexibility, and overall body awareness. It can be adapted to individual fitness

levels and may help address muscle imbalances and posture issues associated with thyroid disorders.

6. Breathing Exercises:
Practicing deep-breathing exercises, such as diaphragmatic breathing or belly breathing, can help manage stress and promote relaxation. Stress reduction is crucial for individuals with thyroid disorders, as stress can impact hormone levels.

7. Interval Training:
High-intensity interval training (HIIT) can be beneficial for individuals seeking efficient workouts. Short bursts of intense exercise followed by rest periods may improve cardiovascular fitness and metabolic rate, supporting overall thyroid health.

8. Swimming:
Swimming is a low-impact exercise that engages multiple muscle groups. It can be gentle on the joints and is suitable for individuals with various fitness levels, providing a well-rounded cardiovascular workout.

9. Mind-Body Practices:
Mind-body practices, such as meditation and guided imagery, contribute to stress reduction and mental well-being. Managing stress is crucial for thyroid health, as chronic stress can impact hormonal balance.

10. Consultation with Healthcare Professionals:
Before starting any exercise regimen, individuals with thyroid disorders should consult with healthcare professionals. They can provide guidance on exercise intensity, duration, and modifications based on individual health conditions.

11. Consistency is Key:
Consistency is essential in any rehabilitation program. Regular, moderate exercise is often more sustainable and beneficial than sporadic intense workouts.

12. Personalized Approach:
Tailoring rehabilitation exercises to individual preferences and needs ensures a personalized and enjoyable fitness routine. Considering individual fitness levels, health goals, and any limitations is crucial for long-term adherence.

In conclusion, rehabilitation exercises and practices can contribute to thyroid health by addressing specific symptoms, promoting overall well-being, and managing stress. It's important to approach exercise mindfully, considering individual needs and consulting with healthcare professionals for personalized guidance.

Yoga, meditation, and mindfulness techniques

Yoga, meditation, and mindfulness techniques are powerful practices that contribute to physical, mental, and emotional well-being. These ancient disciplines offer holistic approaches to managing stress, promoting relaxation, and fostering a sense of balance in modern life.

1. Yoga:

Yoga is a comprehensive system that combines physical postures (asanas), breath control (pranayama), meditation, and ethical principles. The physical postures help improve flexibility, strength, and balance, while the breath control enhances respiratory function. Yoga is known to stimulate the parasympathetic nervous system, promoting relaxation and reducing stress. Certain yoga poses, such as inversions and forward bends, are believed to support thyroid health by stimulating the thyroid gland.

2. Meditation:

Meditation involves cultivating a focused and quiet state of mind, often through mindfulness or concentration techniques. Regular meditation practice has been associated with reduced stress, improved mental clarity, and enhanced emotional well-being. Mindful meditation, in particular, encourages awareness of the present moment, helping individuals manage stressors and maintain a positive outlook.

3. Mindfulness Techniques:

Mindfulness involves paying attention to the present moment without judgment. Techniques such as mindful breathing, body scan, and mindful eating bring awareness to sensations, thoughts, and emotions. Practicing mindfulness can help individuals better cope with stress, anxiety, and negative thought patterns, promoting overall mental resilience.

4. Stress Reduction and Cortisol Management:

Both yoga and meditation are effective tools for reducing cortisol, the stress hormone. Chronic stress can disrupt hormonal balance, including thyroid function. By managing stress, these practices contribute to a healthier hormonal environment.

5. Emotional Regulation:

Mindfulness techniques, including meditation, help individuals observe and regulate their emotions. This emotional self-regulation can positively impact mental health, reducing the risk of conditions such as anxiety and depression.

6. Improved Concentration and Cognitive Function:

Regular practice of yoga, meditation, and mindfulness has been linked to improved cognitive function, including enhanced attention and memory. These practices encourage a state of focused awareness that can translate into better concentration in daily life.

7. Mind-Body Connection:
Yoga, meditation, and mindfulness emphasize the mind-body connection. By fostering awareness of sensations, breath, and movement, individuals can develop a deeper understanding of their bodies and minds, leading to improved overall well-being.

8. Holistic Wellness:
The holistic nature of these practices aligns with a wellness approach that encompasses physical, mental, and emotional dimensions. This holistic perspective recognizes the interconnectedness of various aspects of health and emphasizes balance.

9. Accessible to All:
One of the strengths of yoga, meditation, and mindfulness is their accessibility. These practices can be adapted to different fitness levels, ages, and health conditions, making them inclusive and suitable for a broad range of individuals.

10. Consistent Practice:

Consistency is key for reaping the benefits of yoga, meditation, and mindfulness. Establishing a regular practice, even if for short durations, can lead to cumulative positive effects on overall well-being.

In conclusion, incorporating yoga, meditation, and mindfulness techniques into daily life can be transformative for physical and mental health. These practices offer valuable tools for managing stress, promoting relaxation, and cultivating a mindful approach to life, ultimately contributing to a holistic sense of well-being.

CHAPTER TWENTY-ONE

Alternative healing modalities for

thyroid disorders

Alternative healing modalities encompass a diverse range of approaches that complement conventional medicine and may offer additional support for individuals with thyroid disorders. While alternative therapies are not intended to replace medical treatments, some people find them beneficial as part of an integrative and holistic approach to thyroid health.

1. Acupuncture:
Acupuncture, a traditional Chinese medicine technique, involves the insertion of thin needles into specific points on the body. Some individuals with thyroid disorders explore acupuncture for its potential to reduce stress, improve energy flow, and promote overall well-being.

2. Herbal Medicine:

Herbal remedies, derived from plants, have been used for centuries in traditional healing systems. Adaptogenic herbs like ashwagandha, holy basil, and rhodiola are thought to help the body adapt to stress and may support thyroid function. However, it's crucial to consult with a qualified herbalist or healthcare professional for personalized guidance.

3. Homeopathy:

Homeopathy is based on the principle of "like cures like," using highly diluted substances to stimulate the body's natural healing processes. Some individuals explore homeopathic remedies for symptom management in thyroid disorders. Consulting with a trained homeopath is essential for proper guidance.

4. Mind-Body Practices:

Techniques such as guided imagery, biofeedback, and energy healing practices like Reiki or Qigong aim to balance the body's energy and promote relaxation. These practices may contribute to stress reduction and emotional well-being.

5. Ayurveda:

Ayurveda, an ancient system of medicine from India, emphasizes balancing the body's energies (doshas) through lifestyle, diet, and herbal remedies. Some

Ayurvedic practitioners may recommend specific approaches to support thyroid health based on an individual's dosha.

6. Nutritional Supplements:
Certain nutritional supplements, such as selenium, zinc, and omega-3 fatty acids, are explored by some individuals to support thyroid function. However, it's crucial to approach supplementation cautiously and under the guidance of a healthcare professional to prevent potential interactions or imbalances.

7. Energy Healing:
Practices like energy healing, including practices like Reiki or Healing Touch, focus on the manipulation of energy fields to promote physical and emotional well-being. While anecdotal evidence suggests benefits, scientific validation is limited, and these practices are often considered complementary.

8. Functional Medicine:
Functional medicine explores the root causes of health issues and aims to address imbalances in the body's systems. Some individuals with thyroid disorders seek out functional medicine practitioners who consider factors such as nutrition, lifestyle, and environmental influences.

9. Meditation and Mindfulness:

Mindfulness meditation practices, including Mindfulness-Based Stress Reduction (MBSR), may help manage stress and promote a sense of calm. Stress reduction is crucial for individuals with thyroid disorders, as stress can impact hormone levels.

10. Consultation with Healthcare Professionals:
Before incorporating alternative healing modalities, individuals with thyroid disorders should consult with their healthcare professionals. It's essential to ensure that alternative therapies are safe, do not interfere with prescribed medications, and are suitable for individual health conditions.

In conclusion, alternative healing modalities can be explored by individuals seeking additional support for thyroid health. However, it's crucial to approach these practices mindfully, consult with qualified practitioners, and integrate them as part of a comprehensive and individualized approach to well-being.

Acupuncture, energy healing, and other complementary approaches

Acupuncture, energy healing, and other complementary approaches offer unique perspectives on well-being, often focusing on the interconnectedness of the body's energy systems. While these practices may not replace conventional medical treatments, they can complement traditional approaches and contribute to a holistic understanding of health.

1. Acupuncture:

Acupuncture, rooted in Traditional Chinese Medicine (TCM), involves the insertion of thin needles into specific points on the body to balance the flow of energy or Qi. For individuals with thyroid disorders, acupuncture may be explored to address imbalances in the body's energy and promote overall wellness. Some research suggests that acupuncture may have beneficial effects on thyroid function and stress reduction.

2. Energy Healing:

Energy healing practices, such as Reiki, Healing Touch, and Qigong, work on the premise that disruptions in the body's energy field contribute to illness. Practitioners use various techniques to channel or balance energy, promoting a sense of harmony and facilitating the body's natural healing processes. While scientific evidence is limited, some individuals report positive experiences with energy healing in managing stress and supporting overall well-being.

3. Craniosacral Therapy:

Craniosacral therapy focuses on the manipulation of the membranes and fluids surrounding the brain and spinal cord to enhance the body's self-healing abilities. This gentle, hands-on approach is believed to release tension and improve the functioning of the central nervous system, contributing to overall health and relaxation.

4. Sound Healing:

Sound healing involves the use of vibrational frequencies, such as singing bowls, tuning forks, or vocal toning, to promote relaxation and balance in the body. The vibrations are thought to influence energy flow and may be explored as a complementary practice for stress reduction.

5. Biofield Therapies:

Biofield therapies, including Therapeutic Touch and Healing Touch, focus on working with the body's energy field to promote physical and emotional well-being. Practitioners use gentle hand movements to assess and balance the energy field, aiming to enhance the body's natural healing processes.

6. Magnet Therapy:

Magnet therapy involves the use of magnetic fields to influence the body's energy and promote healing. Some individuals use magnetic devices or wear magnets with the belief that they may have positive effects on energy flow and overall health.

7. Reflexology:

Reflexology is based on the idea that specific points on the hands and feet correspond to different organs and systems in the body. By applying pressure to these points, practitioners aim to stimulate energy flow and promote balance.

8. Mind-Body Practices:

Mind-body practices, including meditation, guided imagery, and breathwork, contribute to stress reduction and overall well-being. These practices acknowledge the mind's influence on the body and encourage a state of relaxation conducive to healing.

9. Consultation with Healthcare Professionals:

Before exploring complementary approaches, individuals should consult with their healthcare professionals, especially if they have thyroid disorders or other medical conditions. Open communication ensures that complementary practices are integrated safely and effectively into an overall health plan.

In conclusion, acupuncture, energy healing, and other complementary approaches offer diverse tools for individuals seeking a holistic approach to well-being. While the scientific evidence supporting these practices varies, many people find value in the mind-body connection and the potential benefits of energy-focused therapies. As with any health-related decisions, an informed and collaborative approach with healthcare professionals is essential for individualized care.

CHAPTER TWENTY-TWO

The connection between thyroid

health and sleep

The connection between thyroid health and sleep is intricate and bidirectional, with thyroid function influencing sleep quality and sleep disturbances impacting thyroid health. The thyroid gland, a crucial part of the endocrine system, plays a central role in regulating metabolism, energy levels, and overall homeostasis. Here's an exploration of how thyroid health and sleep are interconnected:

1. Hypothyroidism and Sleep:
Hypothyroidism, characterized by an underactive thyroid, can contribute to sleep-related issues. Individuals with hypothyroidism may experience fatigue, sluggishness,

and increased need for sleep. The condition can lead to disturbances in sleep patterns, including difficulty falling asleep, frequent awakenings during the night, and overall disrupted sleep architecture.

2. Hyperthyroidism and Sleep:

Conversely, hyperthyroidism, marked by an overactive thyroid, may also affect sleep. Individuals with hyperthyroidism may experience heightened anxiety, restlessness, and increased metabolic activity. These factors can lead to difficulties in initiating and maintaining sleep, resulting in insomnia and sleep deprivation.

3. Sleep Architecture and Hormonal Regulation:

Thyroid hormones, specifically triiodothyronine (T3) and thyroxine (T4), play a role in regulating the body's circadian rhythm and sleep-wake cycle. Disruptions in thyroid function can influence the release and balance of these hormones, impacting the body's ability to enter different stages of sleep, including the restorative stages of deep sleep.

4. Sleep-Related Breathing Disorders:

Thyroid dysfunction may contribute to sleep-related breathing disorders, such as sleep apnea. Changes in thyroid hormone levels can affect respiratory muscles and increase the likelihood of airway obstruction during sleep, leading to disrupted breathing patterns and interruptions in sleep.

5. Impact of Sleep on Thyroid Health:
Conversely, the quality and duration of sleep can influence thyroid function. Sleep deprivation and poor sleep quality may contribute to imbalances in cortisol, a stress hormone that can affect thyroid function. Additionally, disrupted sleep may impact the body's overall ability to regulate and maintain hormonal balance.

6. Addressing Sleep Issues in Thyroid Management:
Addressing sleep issues is an integral part of managing thyroid disorders. Establishing healthy sleep hygiene practices, such as maintaining a consistent sleep schedule, creating a conducive sleep environment, and managing stress, can positively impact both thyroid health and overall well-being.

7. Consultation with Healthcare Professionals:
Individuals experiencing sleep disturbances in conjunction with thyroid disorders should consult with healthcare professionals. Comprehensive evaluation and collaboration with endocrinologists, sleep specialists, and other relevant healthcare providers can help identify and address the specific factors contributing to sleep issues.

In conclusion, the connection between thyroid health and sleep is multifaceted, with thyroid function influencing sleep patterns and sleep disturbances affecting thyroid health. Recognizing and addressing these interrelationships are crucial for individuals managing thyroid disorders, emphasizing the importance of a holistic approach that encompasses both endocrine and sleep health.

Importance of quality sleep for overall well-being

Quality sleep is essential for overall well-being, as it plays a foundational role in supporting physical health, mental clarity, emotional resilience, and optimal daily functioning. The importance of quality sleep cannot be overstated, and its impact extends across various aspects of our lives.

1. Physical Restoration:
During sleep, the body undergoes crucial processes of repair and restoration. Tissues are repaired, muscles are built, and the immune system is strengthened. Quality sleep is integral to maintaining overall physical health, aiding in the recovery from daily wear and tear.

2. Cognitive Function:

Sleep is intricately linked to cognitive function and mental performance. Adequate, restful sleep enhances concentration, memory, and problem-solving skills. It facilitates the consolidation of memories and supports the brain's ability to process information efficiently.

3. Emotional Well-Being:

Quality sleep is closely tied to emotional regulation and resilience. Lack of sleep can contribute to mood swings, increased irritability, and heightened emotional reactivity. On the other hand, sufficient sleep promotes emotional stability, better stress management, and an improved capacity to navigate daily challenges.

4. Hormonal Balance:

Sleep plays a crucial role in maintaining hormonal balance. Disruptions in sleep patterns can impact the release of hormones that regulate appetite, metabolism, and stress response. Consistent, high-quality sleep supports the proper functioning of the endocrine system.

5. Immune System Support:

Sleep is a fundamental component of a healthy immune system. During sleep, the body produces cytokines and other immune system elements that help fight infections and maintain overall immune function. Chronic sleep deprivation can compromise the immune response, making individuals more susceptible to illness.

6. Physical Performance:

For individuals engaged in physical activities or sports, the importance of quality sleep is evident in its impact on physical performance and recovery. Athletes, in particular, benefit from adequate rest to optimize muscle recovery and enhance overall athletic performance.

7. Weight Management:

Quality sleep is associated with healthy weight management. Sleep influences hormones that regulate hunger and satiety. Lack of sleep can disrupt these hormonal signals, leading to increased appetite, cravings for unhealthy foods, and a potential risk of weight gain.

8. Cardiovascular Health:

Consistent, high-quality sleep contributes to cardiovascular health. Sleep helps regulate blood pressure and reduce stress on the cardiovascular system. Chronic sleep deprivation has been linked to an increased risk of cardiovascular issues, including hypertension and heart disease.

9. Mental Health:

The relationship between sleep and mental health is profound. Quality sleep is a protective factor against conditions such as depression, anxiety, and other mood disorders. Addressing sleep patterns is often a crucial component of mental health interventions.

10. Productivity and Daily Functioning:
Overall, the importance of quality sleep is reflected in its positive impact on daily functioning and productivity. Individuals who prioritize and achieve restful sleep are more likely to approach daily tasks with clarity, energy, and efficiency.

In conclusion, quality sleep is a cornerstone of overall well-being, influencing physical health, cognitive function, emotional resilience, and various aspects of daily life. Recognizing the importance of healthy sleep patterns and adopting habits that support restful sleep contribute to a holistic approach to well-being.

Strategies for improving sleep quality with thyroid disorders

Individuals with thyroid disorders often face challenges in maintaining optimal sleep quality due to hormonal imbalances and associated symptoms. Implementing strategies to improve sleep quality is crucial for managing thyroid-related sleep disturbances. Here are effective strategies tailored for individuals with thyroid disorders:

1. Establish a Consistent Sleep Schedule:
Maintain a regular sleep-wake cycle by going to bed and waking up at the same time every day, even on weekends. Consistency reinforces the body's natural circadian rhythm, promoting better sleep quality.

2. Create a Relaxing Bedtime Routine:
Develop a calming pre-sleep routine to signal to your body that it's time to wind down. Activities like reading a book, taking a warm bath, or practicing relaxation techniques can help alleviate stress and prepare the mind for sleep.

3. Optimize Sleep Environment:
Create a comfortable sleep environment by keeping the bedroom cool, dark, and quiet. Invest in a supportive mattress and pillows to enhance physical comfort, and consider using blackout curtains to block out light.

4. Manage Stress and Anxiety:
Stress and anxiety can exacerbate sleep difficulties. Engage in stress-reducing activities such as mindfulness meditation, deep breathing exercises, or gentle yoga to promote relaxation before bedtime.

5. Limit Screen Time Before Bed:

Reduce exposure to electronic devices like phones, tablets, and computers at least an hour before bedtime. The blue light emitted from screens can interfere with the production of the sleep hormone melatonin.

6. Be Mindful of Diet and Timing:
Avoid consuming caffeinated beverages and heavy meals close to bedtime. Stimulants and large meals can disrupt sleep. Instead, opt for a light, balanced snack if needed.

7. Regular Exercise:
Incorporate regular physical activity into your routine, but try to complete exercise sessions at least a few hours before bedtime. Exercise promotes overall well-being and can contribute to better sleep quality.

8. Monitor Thyroid Medications:
Work closely with your healthcare provider to ensure that thyroid medications are optimized and taken at the right time. Adjusting medication dosage or timing may help manage symptoms that affect sleep.

9. Address Sleep Apnea:
Individuals with thyroid disorders may be at an increased risk of sleep apnea. If symptoms such as loud snoring or pauses in breathing are present, consult a healthcare professional for evaluation and potential treatment options.

10. Consult with Healthcare Professionals:

Regular communication with healthcare professionals, including endocrinologists and sleep specialists, is crucial. Discussing sleep difficulties and seeking guidance on potential adjustments to medications or treatments can lead to improved sleep outcomes.

11. Consider Relaxation Techniques:

Incorporate relaxation techniques such as progressive muscle relaxation or guided imagery to calm the mind and body. These practices can be particularly helpful for managing stress-related sleep disturbances.

12. Keep a Sleep Diary:

Maintain a sleep diary to track patterns, sleep quality, and any associated factors. This information can provide valuable insights for healthcare professionals in tailoring interventions to address specific sleep challenges.

In conclusion, adopting a combination of these strategies can contribute to improved sleep quality for individuals with thyroid disorders. Tailoring these approaches to individual preferences and needs, and consulting with healthcare professionals for personalized guidance, ensures a comprehensive and effective approach to managing sleep disturbances associated with thyroid conditions.